The Science of Sleep

The Science of Sleep

Unlocking the Secrets to Restful Nights

Grace Fields

Mindful Pages

Published in 2024

ISBN: 9789358813579 (PB)
ISBN: 9789358813302 (eBook)

Published by

Mindful Pages
Imprint of Alpha Editions LLC
312 W. 2nd St #1834
Casper, WY 82601, USA

The information presented in this book is intended solely for general reading and informational purposes. It is not a substitute for professional medical advice, diagnosis, or treatment.

Please be aware that the content within these pages is not meant to replace the guidance of a registered healthcare professional or doctor. If you have any specific medical concerns, conditions, or questions, you must seek the expertise of a qualified healthcare provider.

Your health and well-being are paramount, and for any medical issue or individual health-related decisions, we strongly advise consulting with a healthcare professional who can provide personalized guidance based on your unique circumstances.

Always prioritize your health and safety, and use this book as a supplementary resource rather than a substitute for professional medical advice.

Contents

Introduction

Welcome to "The Science of Sleep: Unlocking the Secrets to Restful Nights." In our fast-paced, modern lives, sleep is often undervalued and overlooked. We live in a world that glorifies the "work hard, sleep less" mentality as if sleep is an obstacle to success. But the truth is quite the opposite. Sleep is not a hindrance; it's a critical foundation for our overall health and well-being.

Imagine sleep as the architect of our lives, designing and building the framework for our physical and mental health, like a skilled builder, sleep constructs and repairs, ensuring that our bodies and minds are resilient, functional, and ready to face the challenges of each new day.

Picture a day when you've had a truly restful night's sleep. You wake up feeling energized, your mind clear and alert. You're more patient with others, better equipped to make decisions, and resilient in the face of stress. Your body feels agile and pain-free, and your immune system is on high alert, ready to fend off illnesses. You are at your best.

Now, contrast this with a night of restless sleep or chronic sleep deprivation. Your mood is easily irritable, your thoughts foggy, and your reactions slow. Small challenges feel insurmountable, and your body aches. Your immune system is weakened, leaving you susceptible to illnesses. The consequences of inadequate sleep are undeniable.

Why Sleep Matters

Sleep is often seen as a luxury in our modern, fast-paced world, a time-consuming pause in our ceaseless pursuit of productivity and success. We often hear the phrase, "I'll sleep when I'm dead," as if they were postponing sleep as an inconvenience. However, this perspective couldn't be further from the truth. Sleep is not a luxury but a fundamental necessity for our overall health and well-being.

The importance of sleep cannot be overstated. During sleep, our bodies and minds undergo intricate processes essential for survival and vitality. While we slumber, our brains remain active, processing information, consolidating memories, and even engaging in problem-solving.

One of the most critical functions of sleep is physical restoration. While we sleep, our bodies repair and rejuvenate tissues, muscles, and organs. This process is vital for maintaining good health and can be seen in how we feel after a restful night's sleep — refreshed, energized, and ready to tackle the day's challenges.

Moreover, sleep is crucial in regulating our emotions and mental health. A night of insufficient sleep can lead to irritability, mood swings, and heightened stress levels. Chronic sleep deprivation has even been linked to the development of mood disorders such as depression and anxiety. Conversely, adequate sleep can improve emotional resilience and buffer against daily stresses.

Sleep also profoundly influences cognitive functions, including memory, concentration, and problem-solving. During deep sleep, the brain processes and consolidates the information gathered throughout the day. Lack of sleep can impair these functions, making it challenging to focus, learn new things, and make decisions.

Inadequate sleep also takes a toll on our physical health. Numerous studies have linked poor sleep to a higher risk of chronic conditions such as obesity, diabetes, and heart disease. Sleep deprivation can disrupt the balance of hormones that regulate appetite, leading to weight gain, and can contribute to high blood pressure and other cardiovascular issues.

Additionally, sleep is essential for a robust immune system. When we sleep, our bodies produce proteins called cytokines, vital in immune response. Sleep deprivation can compromise our ability to fend off infections, leaving us more susceptible to illnesses.

Sleep isn't just about the quantity of rest we get; it's also about the quality. Achieving restorative sleep involves maintaining a consistent sleep schedule, creating a comfortable sleep environment, and adopting healthy sleep habits. Prioritizing sleep hygiene can lead to more restful nights and improved overall health and well-being.

Sleep is not an inconvenience or a luxury; it is a fundamental requirement for our bodies and minds to function optimally. During sleep, we undergo physical restoration, emotional regulation, and cognitive processing. Neglecting sleep can have profound consequences on our physical and mental health. Therefore, it's time to recognize the importance of sleep and prioritize it as essential to a healthy and fulfilling life. So, the next time you contemplate sacrificing sleep for productivity, remember that sleep matters – it's a precious resource that deserves our attention and respect.

The importance of sleep for overall health and well-being

Sleep is a cornerstone of our existence, often overshadowed by the hustle and bustle of our daily lives. Yet, its importance for overall health and well-being cannot be overstated. Far from being a mere period of inactivity, sleep is a dynamic and essential process that our bodies and minds depend on.

At its core, sleep is a time for rejuvenation. It's when our bodies repair and restore tissues, muscles, and vital organs. This nightly renewal ensures that we wake up refreshed and ready to tackle the day ahead. This rejuvenating process is compromised without adequate sleep, leaving us tired and depleted.

Equally important is sleep's role in emotional regulation. Disrupted or insufficient sleep can result in irritability, mood swings, and heightened stress levels. Over time, chronic sleep deprivation can contribute to the development of mood disorders like depression and anxiety. In contrast, quality sleep fosters emotional resilience, helping us better navigate life's challenges.

Cognitive functions, too, are deeply intertwined with our sleep patterns. While slumbering, our brains actively process and consolidate the information gathered during wakefulness. This includes memory retention, problem-solving, and focusing and learning. Sleep-deprived individuals often struggle with concentration and decision-making, highlighting the importance of restful sleep for mental acuity.

The impact of sleep extends to our physical health. Numerous studies have linked poor sleep to an increased risk of chronic conditions such as obesity, diabetes, and heart disease. Sleep deprivation disrupts the balance of hormones that regulate appetite, often leading to weight gain. It can also contribute to elevated blood pressure and other cardiovascular issues, emphasizing the integral role of sleep in maintaining physical well-being.

Moreover, sleep is a powerful ally in our immune system's fight against infections. During sleep, our bodies produce cytokines, proteins essential for immune response. Insufficient sleep weakens our defences, making us more susceptible to illnesses. A good night's sleep is not merely a luxury but a potent weapon for maintaining a healthy immune system.

In our quest for a healthier and more fulfilling life, we must prioritize sleep as a fundamental building block of overall well-being. This means establishing consistent sleep routines, creating a comfortable sleep environment, and adopting healthy sleep habits. By recognizing the importance of sleep and giving it the attention, it deserves, we can pave the way for improved physical health, emotional balance, and cognitive vitality. In a world that often glorifies sleep deprivation, let us remember that quality sleep is an invaluable asset for achieving our best selves.

In this book, we will embark on an eye-opening journey into the captivating world of sleep science, designed to be accessible to everyone from teenagers to senior citizens. We'll delve into the fundamental aspects of sleep, breaking down complex concepts into simple, understandable terms, and we'll explore how you can harness this knowledge to unlock the secrets to genuinely restful nights.

Sleep doesn't need to be shrouded in mystery, reserved for the experts. Each of us experiences a natural state, typically for a third of our lives. Yet, it's also one of the most underappreciated aspects of human existence. Throughout the following chapters, we'll unravel the science behind sleep, drawing on relatable examples to demystify the sleep cycle, the role of dreams, and the impact of sleep on our physical and mental health.

Whether you're a student trying to balance academics and extracurricular activities, a young adult navigating the demands of a career and family, or an older individual looking to maintain your quality of life as you age, this book is tailored to meet your needs. We all share the common goal of achieving restful nights and waking up refreshed, and by the end of this journey, you'll have a toolbox of knowledge and practical strategies to make it a reality.

So, let's embark on this exploration of sleep together, beginning with the fundamental concepts that underpin this essential aspect of our lives.

1
The Basics of Sleep

Sleep is a fundamental part of our lives, a mysterious realm we enter every night. It's a realm where our bodies and minds undergo profound transformations essential for our daily functioning. In this chapter, we will embark on a journey to unravel the mysteries of sleep, exploring its fundamental elements and how they shape our everyday experiences.

We will ask a simple yet profound question: What is sleep? It's a state we all know intimately, but understanding its intricacies can be enlightening. We'll delve into the different stages of sleep, the sleep-wake cycle, and the role of our internal body clock, the circadian rhythm. By the end of this chapter, you'll have a deeper appreciation for the science behind your nightly adventures in dreamland and how they impact your waking life.

So, let's begin our exploration of the basics of sleep and unlock the secrets within this essential aspect of our existence.

What is Sleep?

Sleep is a remarkable and enigmatic phenomenon that consumes much of our lives. It's a state of altered consciousness, a nightly journey into a realm where the mind wanders and the body rests. But what exactly is sleep, and why is it so crucial for our well-being?

At its core, sleep is a complex and highly orchestrated process orchestrated by our brains. Contrary to the perception that sleep is merely a time of inactivity, it's a period of profound activity within our bodies and minds. When we sleep, we transition through distinct stages, each with unique characteristics and functions.

The sleep cycle consists of two main types of sleep: rapid eye movement (REM) sleep and non-REM sleep. Non-REM sleep is further divided into several stages. As we sleep, we cycle through these stages multiple times at night, each lasting about 90 minutes.

The first stage of non-REM sleep is a transition from wakefulness to sleep. It's a light stage where you may drift in and out of consciousness, and waking up during this phase is relatively easy. As we progress into stage 2, our brain waves slow down, and our heart rate and body temperature drop. This stage prepares us for the deeper stages of sleep.

Stages 3 and 4 are the deep stages of non-REM sleep, also known as slow-wave sleep. During these stages, waking someone up is tricky; if awakened, they may feel dizzy and disoriented. Our bodies engage in physical restoration and repair in these stages. Muscles and tissues are repaired, energy is restored, and growth and immune functions are enhanced.

Then there's REM sleep, which is often associated with vivid dreaming. During REM sleep, our brains become highly active, almost as busy as when awake. However, our bodies become temporarily paralyzed, likely to prevent us from acting out our dreams. REM sleep is essential for cognitive functions like memory consolidation and emotional processing.

So, why do we sleep? The exact purpose of sleep remains a topic of ongoing research and debate among scientists. However, several theories provide insights into its potential functions. One prevalent theory is that sleep plays a crucial role in memory consolidation, allowing our brains to organize and store information acquired throughout the day. This process helps us learn and remember.

Another theory suggests that sleep contributes to physical restoration and repair. During deep non-REM sleep, our bodies release growth hormones, repair tissue, and strengthen the immune system. This may explain why we feel refreshed and revitalized after a good night's sleep.

Sleep also has a role in emotional regulation. A lack of sleep can lead to increased irritability and heightened emotional reactions, while quality sleep can improve our ability to manage stress and maintain a stable mood.

Beyond these functions, sleep's relationship with overall health is well-documented. Adequate sleep is associated with a reduced risk of chronic illnesses such as obesity, diabetes, and heart disease. It also plays a crucial role in immune function, helping us avoid infections.

But sleep is not solely a physical process; it's also influenced by our internal biological clock, known as the circadian rhythm. This internal clock regulates the timing of sleep and wakefulness, controlling when we feel most alert and naturally drowsy.

External cues, most notably light, influence the circadian rhythm. Exposure to natural light during the day and darkness at night helps synchronize our internal clock with the 24-hour day-night cycle. Disrupting this synchronisation in our modern 24/7 society can lead to sleep problems and circadian rhythm disorders.

Circadian rhythms can also shift with age, so teenagers may naturally stay up and wake up later, while older adults tend to become early birds. Understanding these rhythms and aligning our daily routines with them can significantly improve the quality of our sleep.

In summary, sleep is a multifaceted phenomenon encompassing distinct stages, each with its functions. While we may not have all the answers about why we sleep, it's clear that sleep is essential for our physical health, cognitive function, and emotional well-being.

Moreover, our internal biological clock, the circadian rhythm, is pivotal in regulating our sleep-wake cycle. Harnessing the power of this internal clock and prioritizing healthy sleep habits can lead to better sleep quality and overall well-being.

In the hustle and bustle of our lives, it's easy to overlook the importance of sleep, but understanding the intricacies of this vital process reminds us of its significance. So, the next time you close your eyes and drift into slumber, appreciate the incredible journey your body and mind embark on each night—a journey that is indispensable to your health and vitality.

The sleep-wake cycle

The sleep-wake cycle, also known as the circadian rhythm, is a natural, internal process that regulates the timing of sleep and wakefulness over 24 hours. It is driven by our biological clock, which is influenced by external cues like light and temperature. This cycle is essential for maintaining a consistent and healthy sleep pattern.

The sleep-wake cycle consists of two primary phases: the wakefulness phase and the sleep phase, and it helps us adapt to the changing environmental conditions as the day progresses. Here's a breakdown of the sleep-wake cycle:

Wakefulness Phase: This is the period during which we are awake and alert. It typically begins in the morning and lasts until the evening. During this phase, our body temperature and alertness are at their peak. Our energy levels are generally higher, and we are mentally and physically prepared to engage in daily activities.

Sleep Phase: The sleep phase occurs during the nighttime hours when our body transitions into a state of rest and restoration. As the evening progresses, our body temperature decreases, signalling the onset of sleepiness. Our brain produces melatonin, a hormone that helps regulate sleep, making us feel drowsy and facilitating the transition into sleep.

We experience cycles of different sleep stages within the sleep phase, including non-REM (rapid eye movement) and REM sleep. These stages play distinct roles in the restoration of our body and mind. Non-REM sleep is divided into several stages, with stages 3 and 4 being the deepest and most restorative.

Stages 1 and 2: These are the initial stages of non-REM sleep. Stage 1 is a light stage where we can quickly wake up, while stage 2 is a bit deeper. During these stages, our brain waves slow down, decreasing muscle activity.

Stages 3 and 4 are the deep stages of non-REM sleep, also known as slow-wave sleep. During these stages, our brain waves are at their slowest, and waking someone up is difficult. This phase occurs when physical restoration and repair, such as tissue growth and immune system enhancement, is achieved.

REM Sleep: Rapid eye movement (REM) sleep is a unique phase characterized by increased brain activity, vivid dreaming, and temporary muscle paralysis. Although our bodies are relatively immobile during REM sleep, our minds are highly active. It's believed to play a role in memory consolidation and emotional processing.

Our internal body clock regulates the sleep-wake cycle, synchronized with the external environment primarily through exposure to natural light. When we wake up in the morning and get exposure to daylight, it signals our body to suppress melatonin production and become alert. As evening approaches and light diminishes, melatonin levels rise, promoting drowsiness and preparing us for sleep.

Maintaining a consistent sleep-wake schedule is essential to align with our circadian rhythm. Disruptions to this cycle, such as shift work, jet lag, or irregular sleep patterns, can lead to sleep problems and circadian rhythm disorders. These disruptions can result in sleepiness during waking hours, difficulty falling asleep, and sleep disturbances.

Understanding and respecting our natural sleep-wake cycle is crucial for achieving restorative and high-quality sleep. By aligning our daily routines with our circadian rhythm, we can optimize our sleep patterns, improve daily alertness, and enhance overall well-being.

The Circadian Rhythm

External schedules and responsibilities do not solely dictate our lives' daily ebb and flow. Deep within us lies a remarkable and intricate timekeeper known as the circadian rhythm. This internal clock is pivotal in regulating our sleep-wake cycle, influencing our alertness, mood, and overall well-being. Let's embark on a journey to explore this fascinating phenomenon and understand how it profoundly affects our sleep patterns.

What is the Circadian Rhythm?

The term "circadian" is derived from the Latin words "circa" (meaning "around") and "diem" (meaning "day"), and it aptly describes the rhythmic cycle that repeats approximately every 24 hours. The circadian rhythm is, in essence, your body's internal clock that orchestrates various physiological processes and behavioural patterns throughout the day.

The Body's Internal Clock

At the heart of the circadian rhythm lies the suprachiasmatic nucleus (SCN), a tiny cluster of cells in the brain's hypothalamus. This remarkable structure serves as the body's master clock, receiving input from external cues, primarily light, and then relaying this information to various body parts to synchronize their functions.

The Role of Light

Light, particularly natural daylight, is the primary external cue that helps reset and regulate the circadian rhythm. When we wake up and are exposed to sunlight, photoreceptor cells in our eyes send signals to the SCN. This, in turn, triggers the suppression of melatonin, a hormone that makes us feel drowsy and promotes alertness.

As the day progresses and we are exposed to diminishing light, the SCN signals melatonin production, signalling that it's time to prepare for sleep. This natural, daily shift between alertness and drowsiness is integral to the circadian rhythm's influence on our sleep patterns.

How Circadian Rhythm Affects Sleep Patterns

The circadian rhythm profoundly impacts our sleep patterns, determining when we feel most awake and when we are naturally inclined to fall asleep. When our internal clock is in sync with our sleep-wake cycle, we experience optimal sleep quality and wakefulness.

For most individuals, the circadian rhythm aligns with a typical sleep pattern: feeling the most alert and awake during the daytime and progressively drowsier as evening approaches. This natural alignment ensures restorative sleep during the night, thanks to increased melatonin levels.

However, disruptions to our circadian rhythm can result in sleep problems. For example, working night shifts or frequently travelling across time zones can desynchronize our internal clock from the external day-night cycle. This can lead to difficulties falling asleep when needed and feeling excessively tired during waking hours.

Teens often experience shifts in their circadian rhythm, which can cause them to naturally stay up later and struggle to wake up early in the morning. This phenomenon is not simply a matter of preference but is influenced by biological changes that affect their internal clock.

Understanding and respecting your circadian rhythm is crucial for optimizing your sleep patterns. Here are some tips for maintaining a healthy circadian rhythm and improving your sleep:

1. **Maintain a Consistent Sleep Schedule:** Try to go to bed and wake up at the exact times each day, even on weekends. This helps synchronize your internal clock.

2. **Exposure to Natural Light:** Spend time outdoors during daylight hours to reinforce your circadian rhythm's alignment with the external environment.

3. **Limit Exposure to Artificial Light:** Minimize exposure to screens emitting blue light, such as smartphones and computers, in the evening, as it can disrupt your internal clock.

4. **Create a Sleep-Friendly Environment:** Control temperature and noise by making your bedroom comfortable and conducive to sleep.

5. **Practice Good Sleep Hygiene:** Develop healthy sleep habits, such as avoiding caffeine and heavy meals before bedtime.

The circadian rhythm is a remarkable internal clock that governs our sleep-wake cycle and influences our daily functioning. Understanding its role in our lives and aligning our routines with natural patterns can improve sleep quality, enhance alertness, and enhance overall well-being. It reminds us that, just as the natural world operates in rhythmic cycles, so do our bodies, and respecting these cycles can be the key to a healthier and more harmonious life.

2
The Physiology of Sleep

As we delve deeper into the world of sleep, our journey takes us into the intricate realm of sleep physiology. This chapter explores the remarkable processes that unfold within our bodies and minds during those precious hours of slumber. Understanding the physiology of sleep is like peeling back the layers of a fascinating mystery, revealing the hidden mechanisms that govern our rest and restoration.

We will uncover the astonishing transformations during sleep, from synchronizing brain activity to rejuvenating our physical form. It's a journey that will shed light on why we need sleep, how our bodies regulate it, and how it contributes to our well-being.

So, let us embark on this voyage into the physiology of sleep, where the science of rest meets the art of rejuvenation.

Brain Activity During Sleep: Unraveling the Secrets of Our Nocturnal Minds

Sleep is far from being a passive state of rest. It's a complex and dynamic process involving remarkable brain activity changes, orchestrated by an intricate symphony of neural rhythms and hormonal signals. In this exploration, we will delve into the inner workings of our brains during sleep, uncovering the fascinating details of brain waves during different sleep stages and the crucial role played by the pineal gland and melatonin in regulating our nocturnal journey.

Understanding Brain Waves During Different Sleep Stages

The sleep journey is marked by distinct phases, each characterized by unique patterns of brain activity. Electroencephalography (EEG) has allowed scientists to peer into the minds of slumbering individuals and decipher these cerebral symphonies.

Wakefulness and Stage 1 Sleep: When we are awake and alert, our brains generate beta waves, which are fast and desynchronized. As we transition into sleep, particularly during the early stages of drowsiness, our brain waves shift to alpha waves, signalling relaxation. Stage 1 sleep is a transitional phase marked by theta waves. These waves are slower and less regular, often accompanied by fleeting, dream-like thoughts.

Stage 2 Sleep: This is a deeper stage of sleep, characterized by the emergence of sleep spindles and K-complexes. Sleep spindles are brief bursts of fast, rhythmic brain waves, while K-complexes are sharp, high-amplitude waves. These patterns play a role in protecting sleep from disruptions, such as external noises.

Stages 3 and 4 (Slow-Wave Sleep): These are the deepest stages of non-REM sleep, distinguished by slow delta waves. Delta waves are large and synchronized, representing the most profound form of restorative sleep. During these stages, the body undergoes physical repair and growth while the mind consolidates memory.

REM Sleep: Rapid eye movement (REM) sleep is a phase of heightened brain activity characterized by desynchronized, rapid, and irregular brain waves similar to wakefulness. It's during REM sleep that vivid dreaming occurs. Despite the brain's high activity, the body's muscles are temporarily paralyzed, likely to prevent us from acting out our dreams.

Role of the Pineal Gland and Melatonin

The pineal gland, a tiny pinecone-shaped structure deep within the brain, is pivotal in regulating our sleep-wake cycle. One of its primary functions is to produce melatonin, a hormone that helps synchronize our internal body clock with the day-night cycle.

Melatonin Production: The pineal gland produces melatonin in response to diminishing light levels, primarily in the evening—this surge in melatonin signals to the body that it's time to prepare for sleep. Melatonin levels remain elevated throughout the night, promoting restful slumber.

As morning light increases, melatonin production wanes, gradually awakening the body.

Circadian Rhythm Synchronization: Melatonin is crucial in regulating our circadian rhythm. Exposure to light, particularly natural daylight, suppresses melatonin production, signalling to the body that it's time to be alert and awake. Conversely, the absence of light triggers melatonin release, facilitating sleepiness and promoting restorative sleep.

Melatonin Supplements: Melatonin supplements are sometimes used to address sleep disorders, particularly those related to circadian rhythm disruptions, such as jet lag or shift work. These supplements can help realign the internal body clock with the external environment.

Understanding the intricate dance of brain waves during different sleep stages and the role of the pineal gland and melatonin in regulating our sleep-wake cycle provides us with profound insights into sleep physiology. It underscores the importance of maintaining a consistent sleep schedule, managing exposure to artificial light in the evening, and nurturing a sleep-friendly environment to support healthy sleep patterns.

Sleep is a marvel of nature, a realm where our brains orchestrate intricate neural rhythms and hormone symphonies. The phases of sleep, marked by evolving brain wave patterns, ensure our physical and mental restoration. With its melatonin production, the pineal gland acts as a conductor, synchronizing our internal body clock with the natural cadence of day and night. As we unravel the mysteries of brain activity during sleep, we gain a deeper appreciation for the profound importance of restful slumber in our lives.

The Sleep Architecture: Unraveling the Blueprint of a Restful Night

Sleep, that nightly voyage into the realm of dreams and rejuvenation, is far from a monotonous state of unconsciousness. It is, in fact, a finely choreographed performance by our brains and bodies, with distinct phases and patterns that collectively form the blueprint of our sleep architecture. This exploration will explore the intricacies of sleep cycles, their significance, and the fascinating realms of REM (Rapid Eye Movement) sleep and non-REM sleep.

Sleep Cycles and Their Significance

Sleep is not a static state but a dynamic one characterized by cyclical patterns of brain activity and physiological changes. These cycles are instrumental in orchestrating the various processes that occur during sleep.

The Sleep Cycle

The fundamental unit of sleep architecture is the sleep cycle, which typically lasts about 90 minutes and repeats throughout the night. A complete sleep cycle consists of two main categories of sleep: REM (Rapid Eye Movement) and non-REM sleep. These categories can be further divided into distinct stages, each with unique characteristics.

Non-REM Sleep (NREM)

Stage 1: The journey begins with the transition from wakefulness to sleep. In Stage 1, you're in a light sleep, easily awakened. Brain activity slows, and you may experience fleeting, dream-like thoughts.

Stage 2: As you proceed deeper into sleep, Stage 2 is where you spend a significant portion of your night. During this phase, brain waves become slower, and sleep spindles—brief bursts of fast, rhythmic brain activity—and K-complexes protect against external disruptions.

Stages 3 and 4 (Slow-Wave Sleep): These stages of deep, slow-wave sleep, where delta waves—large, synchronized, and slow brain waves—predominate. This is the most vital phase of sleep, associated with physical repair, growth, and immune system enhancement.

REM Sleep (Rapid Eye Movement)

After cycling through non-REM sleep, you enter the fascinating realm of REM sleep, characterized by a paradoxical combination of heightened brain activity and muscle paralysis.

Vivid Dreaming: REM sleep is the stage where vivid dreaming occurs. Your brain is nearly as active as when you're awake, and your eyes dart rapidly beneath closed lids—hence the name Rapid Eye Movement.

Muscle Paralysis: While your mind is intensely active, your body remains almost completely paralyzed during REM sleep. This muscle paralysis is believed to prevent us from physically acting out our dreams.

The significance of these sleep cycles lies in their role in memory consolidation, emotional processing, and physical restoration. Non-REM sleep, particularly the deep stages, is crucial for physical health, while REM sleep plays a pivotal role in cognitive and emotional well-being.

REM (Rapid Eye Movement) Sleep and Non-REM Sleep

Non-REM Sleep: The Body's Restoration Workshop

Non-REM sleep is often described as the "restorative" phase, encompassing stages 1 through 4. The body engages in essential physical recovery and maintenance processes during this time.

Physical Repair: Stages 3 and 4, characterized by slow-wave sleep, are the periods of deep physical restoration. Tissue repair, muscle growth, and the release of growth hormones all occur during these stages.

Immune System Enhancement: Slow-wave sleep also bolsters the immune system, enhancing its ability to fend off infections and diseases. Adequate slow-wave sleep is vital for maintaining overall health.

Memory Consolidation: Non-REM sleep, particularly Stage 2, plays a role in memory consolidation. It helps organize and store the information gathered during the day, facilitating learning and memory retention.

REM (Rapid Eye Movement) Sleep: The Theater of Dreams

REM sleep, on the other hand, is the enigmatic stage of sleep marked by heightened brain activity and vivid dreaming. Despite the absence of physical movement, this phase is mentally active and emotionally charged.

Dreaming: REM sleep is the stage where dreams are most vivid and emotionally charged. These dreams serve various functions, including emotional processing, problem-solving, and memory consolidation.

Cognitive Benefits: REM sleep contributes to cognitive functions such as creativity and problem-solving. It allows the brain to process and make sense of emotions and experiences.

Learning and Memory: REM sleep has a role in learning and memory consolidation, complementing the functions of non-REM sleep. It helps organize and store information gathered during waking hours.

In conclusion, sleep architecture is a mesmerizing blueprint that guides us through the night, encompassing sleep cycles, non-REM sleep, and REM sleep.

3

The Sleep Environment

In the quest for restful and rejuvenating sleep, we often focus on the science of slumber—understanding the intricacies of sleep cycles, brain activity, and hormonal regulation. While these factors undoubtedly play a crucial role, we must not overlook a fundamental element that can significantly impact the quality of our sleep: the sleep environment.

Our sleep environment is the stage upon which our nightly performance unfolds, and its design and ambience can either support or hinder our journey into dreamland. In this chapter, we will explore the importance of crafting the ideal sleep environment—a sanctuary where the conditions are optimized for peaceful and restorative sleep.

The sleep environment encompasses a range of factors that collectively shape the quality of our slumber. It includes elements such as lighting, temperature, noise levels, bedding, and even the arrangement of furniture within our bedrooms. Each of these elements can profoundly influence the ease with which we fall asleep, the duration of our rest, and the overall quality of our sleep.

Consider, for instance, the impact of lighting. Exposure to natural light during the day helps regulate our circadian rhythm, synchronizing our internal clock with the external day-night cycle. Conversely, excessive artificial light, particularly in the evening, can disrupt this delicate balance, making it harder to fall asleep and stay asleep. By optimizing the lighting in our sleep environment, we can better support our body's natural sleep-wake cycle.

Temperature is another critical element. A bedroom that is too warm or cold can interfere with our comfort and the body's ability to regulate its temperature during sleep. Maintaining a comfortably cool room temperature can promote restful slumber, as our bodies naturally cool when we sleep.

Noise levels in the sleep environment can also impact sleep quality. External noises like traffic or neighbours can disrupt our sleep patterns. Creating a quiet space or using white noise machines can help mask disruptive sounds, allowing us to sleep more soundly.

Bedding and mattress quality play a pivotal role in our sleep experience. An uncomfortable mattress or unsupportive pillow can lead to aches, pains, and discomfort during the night. Choosing the suitable bedding materials and mattress firmness can significantly affect our overall sleep comfort.

Furthermore, the arrangement and organization of our bedrooms can contribute to a sense of calm and relaxation. Clutter and disarray can create stress and anxiety, making it challenging to unwind and fall asleep. Maintaining a tidy and harmonious sleep environment can foster a sense of tranquillity conducive to restful nights.

Crafting the perfect sleep environment is a deeply personal endeavour. What works for one individual may not work for another, as our preferences and sensitivities vary. Tailoring your sleep environment to your specific needs and preferences is essential.

In the following sections of this chapter, we will delve into each element of the sleep environment in greater detail, offering tips and strategies to optimize your sleep sanctuary. From creating the ideal lighting conditions to selecting the perfect bedding and regulating temperature, we will provide insights and guidance to help you craft a sleep environment that promotes restful and restorative sleep.

The journey into the heart of the sleep environment is an exploration of the art of sleep. It is an acknowledgement of our surroundings' profound impact on the quality of our sleep and, by extension, our overall health and well-being. As we embark on this journey, let us be mindful of the transformative power of a thoughtfully designed sleep environment that nurtures our dreams and supports our quest for restful nights.

Creating a Sleep-Friendly Bedroom

Creating a sleep-friendly bedroom is pivotal in fostering restful and rejuvenating nights. This sacred space serves as the backdrop for our nightly journey into the realm of dreams, where we seek solace and renewal. To optimize your sleep environment, consider the elements contributing to a soothing and tranquil bedroom.

Lighting plays a pivotal role in creating the right ambience for sleep. Natural light during the day helps regulate your body's internal clock, so use blackout curtains to block out external light sources and ensure a dark and restful environment at night. Soft, warm lighting creates a cosy atmosphere, while harsh, bright lights disrupt your sleep-wake cycle.

Temperature control is essential for comfort during sleep. A bedroom that's too hot or cold can lead to restless nights. Finding the right balance by adjusting your thermostat or using appropriate bedding materials can help create a sleep-conducive temperature.

The quality of your mattress and bedding greatly influences your sleep experience. An uncomfortable mattress or unsupportive pillows can lead to aches and pains, making it challenging to drift into slumber. Invest in bedding that suits your comfort preferences and promotes restful sleep.

Noise levels can significantly impact your ability to fall asleep and stay asleep. Consider using white noise machines or earplugs to mask disruptive sounds, ensuring a quieter sleep environment. Alternatively, you can incorporate soothing sounds, like gentle rainfall or ocean waves, to create a calming audio backdrop.

Organization and clutter control plays a crucial role in the tranquillity of your sleep space. A cluttered and disorganized bedroom can lead to feelings of stress and anxiety. Maintain a tidy and organized room to promote a sense of calm and relaxation.

Your bedroom's colour scheme and decor can influence your mood and sleep quality. Choose calming colours like soft blues, gentle greens, or muted earth tones to create a serene atmosphere. Avoid bright, vibrant colours that may be too stimulating for a sleep-friendly environment.

Consider the arrangement of your furniture within the bedroom. Ensure that the layout promotes relaxation and ease of movement. Create a harmonious flow that encourages a sense of tranquillity.

Electronics like televisions, computers, and smartphones emit blue light, which can interfere with your circadian rhythm. Limiting or eliminating these devices from your bedroom is advisable to minimize disruptions to your sleep-wake cycle.

Finally, personal touches and sensory elements can enhance your sleep environment. Incorporate soothing scents like lavender or chamomile through essential oils or candles. Soft, breathable fabrics for your bedding and curtains can provide a tactile sense of comfort.

Creating a sleep-friendly bedroom is a deeply personal endeavour. Your preferences and sensitivities will dictate your choices in designing this sanctuary for rest. Paying attention to the elements contributing to a peaceful and soothing sleep environment can pave the way for restful nights and a more vibrant waking life.

Tips for optimizing your sleep environment

Control Lighting: Use blackout curtains to block out external light sources, and consider installing dimmer switches for adjustable bedroom lighting. Avoid exposure to bright screens (e.g., smartphones and computers) before bedtime, as the blue light can disrupt your sleep-wake cycle.

Maintain a Comfortable Temperature: Keep your bedroom at a temperature that suits your comfort preferences. A more relaxed room is generally more conducive to sleep, but find the best temperature for you. Use appropriate bedding materials like blankets and sheets to regulate temperature.

Invest in a Quality Mattress and Bedding: Choose a mattress and pillows that provide your body the proper support and comfort. High-quality bedding materials can enhance your sleep experience.

Manage Noise Levels: Use white noise machines, earplugs, or soothing sounds (like nature sounds or calming music) to mask disruptive noises. Alternatively, you can create a quiet environment by soundproofing your bedroom.

Declutter and Organize: A tidy and organized bedroom promotes a sense of calm and relaxation. Keep your sleeping space clutter-free to minimize stress and anxiety.

Select Calming Colours and Decor: Choose calming colours like soft blues, gentle greens, or muted earth tones for your bedroom walls and decor. Avoid bright and vibrant colours that may be too stimulating.

Arrange Furniture for Flow: Arrange your bedroom furniture to create a harmonious flow that encourages relaxation and ease of movement. Ensure that the layout promotes a sense of tranquillity.

Limit Electronics: Minimize or eliminate electronics, such as televisions, computers, and smartphones, from your bedroom. These devices emit blue light that can disrupt your circadian rhythm.

Add Personal Touches: Incorporate sensory elements like soothing scents (through essential oils or candles) and soft, breathable fabrics for bedding and curtains. These personal touches can enhance your sleep environment.

Maintain a Clean Air Quality: Ensure your bedroom has good air circulation and is allergens-free. Use air purifiers or open windows, when possible, to maintain clean air quality.

Create a Comfortable Sleep Schedule: Establish a consistent sleep schedule by going to bed and waking up at the exact times every day, even on weekends. This helps regulate your body's internal clock.

Optimise Comfort: Invest in a comfortable mattress, pillows, and bedding that align with your preferences for firmness and softness.

Minimise Light and Sound: Use blackout curtains to block out external light sources, and consider using earplugs or a white noise machine to minimize disruptive sounds.

Temperature Control: To promote restful sleep, keep your bedroom comfortable, typically cooler rather than warmer. Use blankets and layers that you can adjust as needed.

Remove Electronics: Remove or limit the presence of electronic devices like TVs, computers, and smartphones in the bedroom to reduce exposure to blue light and potential sleep disruptions.

Soothing Scents: Use aromatherapy with calming scents like lavender or chamomile to create a relaxing atmosphere.

Comfortable Bedding: Invest in comfortable, high-quality bedding that suits your sleep preferences, including pillows and mattress toppers.

Optimise Bedding: Choose bedding materials that promote temperature regulation, such as moisture-wicking sheets or cooling mattress pads.

Minimise Allergens: Keep your bedroom clean and dust-free to minimize allergens that can disrupt sleep and trigger allergies.

Personal Touches: Add personal touches like photos, artwork, or soothing decorations that make your bedroom a welcoming and comfortable space.

By implementing these tips, you can transform your bedroom into a sleep-friendly sanctuary that promotes restful and rejuvenating nights, ultimately improving your overall well-being.

The Importance of Comfortable Bedding and Temperature for Restful Sleep

A restful night's sleep is a precious commodity, and its quality often hinges on two key factors: comfortable bedding and the right sleep temperature. These elements are fundamental to creating a sleep-friendly environment that promotes relaxation, minimizes disruptions, and enhances the overall sleep experience.

The Quest for Comfortable Bedding

The relationship between comfortable bedding and quality sleep is undeniable. Your choice of mattress, pillows, sheets, and blankets can significantly impact how you rest. Here's why comfortable bedding matters:

1. Support and Alignment

A quality mattress provides the necessary support to maintain proper spinal alignment, alleviating pressure points and preventing discomfort or pain during the night. The right level of support promotes healthy sleep posture, reducing the risk of waking up with aches and pains.

2. Temperature Regulation

Comfortable bedding materials help regulate your body temperature, a critical factor in sleep quality. Breathable sheets, moisture-wicking fabrics, and cooling mattress toppers can prevent overheating and night sweats, contributing to uninterrupted sleep.

3. Reduced Allergen Exposure

Hypoallergenic bedding materials, like dust mite-resistant covers and anti-allergen pillows, can minimize allergen exposure, which can otherwise lead to allergies or exacerbate existing respiratory issues, disrupting sleep.

4. Customized Comfort

Pillows, mattress toppers, and blankets come in various materials and firmness levels, allowing you to customize your sleep environment to suit your preferences. Whether you prefer the plush embrace of memory foam or the support of a firm mattress, tailored bedding ensures your comfort.

5. Psychological Comfort

Comfortable bedding provides a psychological sense of security and relaxation. The tactile pleasure of soft sheets and the cosy embrace of a warm blanket signal to your brain that it's time to unwind, promoting a restful state of mind.

The Crucial Role of Temperature

Temperature, both room temperature and your body's temperature, plays a pivotal role in sleep quality:

1. Sleep Environment Temperature

Maintaining a comfortable room temperature is essential for sleep. A more fantastic room (around 65-70°F or 18-21°C) is generally conducive to restful slumber. Cooler temperatures help your body reach its optimal sleep temperature, reducing the likelihood of night sweats and restlessness.

2. Temperature Regulation

Your body temperature naturally drops as you prepare for sleep. Adequate temperature control in your sleep environment supports this process. Excellent rooms and breathable bedding materials help regulate temperature, allowing your body to enter more profound and therapeutic sleep stages.

3. Comfort and Relaxation

A comfortable sleep environment temperature contributes to a sense of relaxation. Feeling too hot or too cold can create discomfort and awaken you during the night. Maintaining an optimal sleep temperature promotes uninterrupted sleep.

4. Circadian Rhythm Alignment

A consistent sleep environment temperature helps synchronize your internal body clock (circadian rhythm) with the external day-night cycle. Exposure to cooler temperatures in the evening signals to your body that it's time to prepare for sleep.

5. Reduced Nighttime Awakenings

Extreme temperatures in either direction can lead to nighttime awakenings. A hot room may cause night sweats and discomfort, while a chilly room can lead to waking up feeling too cold. Maintaining the right sleep temperature minimizes disruptions.

In conclusion, comfortable bedding and the right sleep temperature are integral to a restful night's sleep. They support physical and psychological comfort, help regulate body temperature, and reduce sleep quality disruptions. Investing in quality bedding materials and maintaining an optimal sleep environment temperature can go a long way in ensuring that each night's sleep is a rejuvenating and refreshing experience.

Sleep Hygiene

Sleep hygiene refers to habits and practices promoting good sleep quality and overall sleep health. Like personal hygiene routines for maintaining physical cleanliness, sleep hygiene is a series of behaviours and environmental factors to optimize sleep duration and quality. Good sleep hygiene is essential for achieving restorative sleep, improving daytime alertness, and preventing sleep disorders. This article will delve into the critical components of sleep hygiene and why they are crucial for a healthy sleep pattern.

Consistent Sleep Schedule

One of the fundamental principles of sleep hygiene is maintaining a consistent sleep schedule. This means going to bed and waking up simultaneously every day, even on weekends. Your body has an internal circadian rhythm, which regulates sleep-wake cycles. Consistency reinforces this natural rhythm, helping your body anticipate sleep and wake times. Irregular sleep patterns can lead to circadian rhythm disruptions, making falling asleep and waking up at desired times challenging.

Create a Comfortable Sleep Environment

The sleep environment plays a crucial role in sleep quality. To enhance sleep hygiene, creating a comfortable sleep environment is essential. Factors to consider include:

Comfortable Bed and Bedding: Invest in a comfortable mattress and pillows that suit your preferences for firmness and softness. High-quality bedding materials can also contribute to better sleep.

Optimal Room Temperature: Maintain a room temperature conducive to sleep, typically on the cooler side (around 65-70°F or 18-21°C). Cooler temperatures support the body's natural cooling process during sleep.

Darkness and Quiet: Block out external light sources using blackout curtains and minimize noise disruptions using earplugs or white noise machines. A dark and quiet environment promotes restful sleep.

Limit Electronics: Remove or reduce the presence of electronic devices, such as televisions, computers, and smartphones, in the bedroom. These devices emit blue light, disrupting your circadian rhythm and making it difficult to fall asleep.

Maintain a Relaxing Bedtime Routine

Establishing a relaxing bedtime routine signals your body that it's time to wind down and prepare for sleep. This routine can include reading, taking a warm bath, practising relaxation techniques, or gentle stretching exercises. Avoid stimulating activities like watching thrilling movies or engaging in intense exercise right before bedtime, as these can make it harder to fall asleep.

Be Mindful of Diet and Hydration

What you eat and drink can significantly impact your sleep. It's important to avoid heavy or spicy meals close to bedtime, as they can cause discomfort and indigestion. Additionally, limit caffeine and alcohol intake in the hours leading up to bedtime, as these substances can interfere with sleep patterns. Staying hydrated is essential, but avoid excessive liquids right before bedtime to minimize nighttime awakenings to use the bathroom.

Regular Physical Activity

Regular physical activity can improve sleep quality, but it's essential to time your exercise appropriately. Engaging in vigorous physical activity too close to bedtime can be stimulating and make it harder to fall asleep. Aim to complete your exercise routine at least a few hours before bedtime to allow your body to relax.

Manage Stress and Anxiety

Stress and anxiety are common culprits of sleep disturbances. Practising stress-reduction techniques, such as mindfulness meditation, deep breathing exercises, or progressive muscle relaxation, can help calm your mind and reduce the impact of stress on your sleep.

Sleep hygiene encompasses practices and behaviours essential for maintaining healthy sleep patterns and optimizing sleep quality. Adopting these habits and creating a conducive sleep environment can enhance your sleep hygiene and allow you to enjoy more restful and rejuvenating nights. Prioritizing sleep hygiene is a valuable step toward achieving better overall health and well-being through improved sleep.

4
Sleep Disorders

While sleep is often viewed as a nightly journey into the realm of dreams and rejuvenation, it remains an enigmatic and elusive experience for many. In the previous chapters, we explored the art and science of sleep, from the essentials of sleep physiology to the importance of a sleep-friendly environment. Now, we embark on a journey into the world of sleep disorders—a landscape where turbulent currents can disrupt sleep's tranquil shores.

Sleep disorders are a diverse and complex group of conditions that affect millions of individuals worldwide. These disorders encompass a broad spectrum, from difficulties falling asleep and staying asleep to behaviours and movements during sleep that can be fascinating and perplexing. They can disrupt not only the quantity of sleep one receives but also the quality, leading to daytime fatigue, impaired functioning, and a diminished quality of life.

This chapter will illuminate the various sleep disorders that plague our nights, exploring their causes, symptoms, and potential treatments. From common disorders like insomnia and sleep apnea to rarer conditions like parasomnias and restless legs syndrome, we will delve into the intricate tapestry of sleep disruptions that can affect individuals of all ages.

Sleep disorders are more than just inconveniences—genuine medical concerns warranting attention and intervention. They can impact physical health, mental well-being, and overall quality of life. Yet, understanding these disorders is the first step toward managing and overcoming them.

As we navigate the terrain of sleep disorders, we will uncover the fascinating complexities of sleep that lie beneath the surface. We will learn how disturbances in sleep architecture and neural signalling can give rise to conditions that range from mild to severe. Most importantly, we will explore diagnosis, treatment, and prevention strategies, empowering individuals to reclaim their nights and enjoy the therapeutic benefits of restful slumber.

So, let us embark on this journey into sleep disorders. This journey will unveil the mysteries of sleep disruptions and offer insights into the path to peaceful, uninterrupted rest.

Common Sleep Disorders

Sleep is a universal necessity, an essential aspect of human biology and physiology. Yet, for many, sleeping remains elusive, fraught with challenges that disrupt the natural rhythm of rest. Common sleep disorders stand as formidable adversaries to the tranquillity of slumber, affecting millions of people worldwide. In this exploration, we venture into the world of these sleep disturbances, unveiling the complexities that underlie their prevalence and impact on individuals' lives.

Sleep disorders encompass various conditions that interfere with sleep initiation, maintenance, and quality. From the restless tossing and turning of insomnia to the breathless pauses of sleep apnea, these disorders can manifest in various forms, affecting people of all ages, genders, and backgrounds.

Understanding these common sleep disorders is paramount for those who experience them, healthcare providers, researchers, and anyone interested in the fascinating intersection of sleep and health. Sleep is a fundamental pillar of well-being, and disruptions can have far-reaching consequences.

Further, we will shine a light on each sleep disorder, uncovering the intricacies of their symptoms and diagnostic criteria. We will explore the potential risk factors contributing to their development and the various treatment options available to help individuals regain sleep control.

Sleep is vital to our lives, and its disorders should not be taken lightly. They can affect our physical health, cognitive function, emotional well-being, and overall quality of life. By gaining insights into these common sleep disorders, we can bridge the gap between restless nights and refreshing slumber, offering hope and solutions to those seeking reprieve from disrupted sleep's challenges.

Join us on this journey into the world of common sleep disorders as we unravel the mysteries that lurk in the darkness of restless nights and pave the way toward a future of peaceful, rejuvenating sleep.\

Common Sleep Disorders

1. Insomnia:

Symptoms:

- Difficulty falling asleep
- Frequent awakenings during the night
- Waking up too early and being unable to fall back asleep
- Non-restorative sleep, leading to daytime fatigue
- Irritability, mood disturbances, and impaired concentration

Causes:

- Stress and anxiety
- Depression
- Medical conditions or chronic pain
- Medications
- Poor sleep habits
- Shift work or irregular sleep schedules
- Lifestyle factors, such as excessive caffeine or alcohol consumption

Treatment Options:

- Cognitive-behavioural therapy for insomnia (CBT-I)
- Medications, including sedatives or hypnotics (prescribed by a healthcare professional)
- Addressing underlying medical or psychological conditions
- Improving sleep hygiene and creating a sleep-conducive environment
- Stress reduction techniques, relaxation exercises, and mindfulness meditation

2. Sleep Apnea:

Symptoms:

- Loud, chronic snoring
- Episodes of breathing cessation during sleep
- Gasping or choking sounds during sleep
- Excessive daytime sleepiness
- Morning headaches
- Difficulty concentrating and irritability
- Decreased libido

Causes:

- Obstructive sleep apnea (OSA): Occurs when throat muscles relax excessively, leading to a blocked airway.
- Central sleep apnea: Results from the brain's failure to send appropriate signals to the muscles controlling breathing.
- Complex sleep apnea syndrome: A combination of OSA and central sleep apnea.

Treatment Options:

- Continuous Positive Airway Pressure (CPAP) therapy: This device delivers a continuous stream of air to keep the airway open.
- Bilevel Positive Airway Pressure (BiPAP) therapy Provides variable pressure for inhalation and exhalation.
- Lifestyle changes, such as weight loss and avoiding alcohol and sedatives
- Positional therapy (encouraging side sleeping)
- Surgery to remove or reposition excess tissue or correct structural issues (in severe cases)

3. Restless Leg Syndrome (RLS):

Symptoms:

- Uncomfortable sensations in the legs, often described as creeping, crawling, or tingling

- An irresistible urge to move the legs, typically worsened by rest or inactivity

- Symptoms that are relieved temporarily by movement

- Sleep disturbances and daytime fatigue

Causes:

- The exact cause is unknown, but genetics may play a role.

- Iron deficiency or anaemia

- Chronic diseases, such as kidney failure, diabetes, or peripheral neuropathy

- Pregnancy-related hormonal changes

- Medications, including certain antipsychotics and antidepressants

Treatment Options:

- Lifestyle modifications, such as regular exercise and maintaining a consistent sleep schedule

- Iron supplementation (if an iron deficiency is detected)

- Medications that can help alleviate symptoms, including dopamine agonists, anticonvulsants, and opioids (prescribed by a healthcare professional)

- Management of any underlying medical conditions

- Avoidance of caffeine and alcohol, which can exacerbate symptoms

These are just a few common sleep disorders, each with unique symptoms, causes, and treatment options. It's essential to consult with a healthcare professional for a proper diagnosis and personalized treatment plan if you suspect you may be experiencing a sleep disorder.

Sleep Disorders and Their Impact

Sleep disorders, often concealed in the darkness of restless nights, can significantly influence overall health and quality of life. These disorders encompass a broad spectrum of conditions, from insomnia and sleep apnea to restless leg syndrome and narcolepsy. While they may vary in their symptoms and causes, their potential impact on physical health, mental well-being, and overall quality of life should not be underestimated.

How Sleep Disorders Affect Overall Health and Quality of Life

1. **Daytime Fatigue and Impaired Functioning:** One of the most immediate consequences of sleep disorders is daytime fatigue. Individuals with sleep disorders often struggle to maintain alertness, focus, and productivity during waking hours. This can impact work performance, academic achievements, and overall functioning in daily life.

2. **Mental Health Implications:** Sleep and mental health are closely intertwined. Sleep disorders can exacerbate or contribute to conditions like anxiety, depression, and mood disorders. In some cases, they may even trigger or worsen symptoms of existing mental health conditions.

3. **Physical Health Risks:** Several sleep disorders, such as sleep apnea, have been linked to significant physical health risks. Sleep apnea, for example, can increase the risk of hypertension, heart disease, stroke, and diabetes. Sleep disorders can also compromise the immune system, making individuals more susceptible to illness.

4. **Weight Gain and Metabolic Dysregulation:** Poor sleep patterns, often associated with sleep disorders, can disrupt the body's hunger-regulating hormones. This can lead to overeating, weight gain, and an increased risk of metabolic disorders like obesity and type 2 diabetes.

5. **Decreased Quality of Life:** The cumulative impact of sleep disorders on various aspects of life, including relationships, leisure activities, and social interactions, can lead to a diminished overall quality of life. The constant

struggle to achieve restorative sleep can erode one's sense of well-being and contentment.

The Role of Genetics in Sleep Disorders

While lifestyle factors and environmental influences certainly play a role in sleep disorders, genetics also contribute significantly to their development and prevalence. The interplay between genetic factors and sleep disorders can be observed in several ways:

1. **Family History:** A family history of sleep disorders, such as insomnia or sleep apnea, can increase an individual's susceptibility to these conditions. Shared genetic traits within families can predispose multiple members to similar sleep-related challenges.

2. **Genetic Variants:** Specific genetic variants are associated with certain sleep disorders. For instance, gene variations related to circadian rhythms can influence an individual's natural sleep-wake cycle and susceptibility to conditions like delayed sleep phase disorder.

3. **Hereditary Conditions:** Some sleep disorders have a hereditary component. Restless leg syndrome, for example, tends to run in families, suggesting a genetic link.

4. **Response to Treatment:** Genetic differences can influence how individuals respond to various treatments for sleep disorders. Understanding these genetic variations can help healthcare providers tailor treatment approaches to individual patients.

Sleep disorders are not isolated disturbances but rather complex conditions with far-reaching consequences. They impact the quantity and quality of sleep and extend their effects into physical and mental health, social well-being, and overall life satisfaction. While genetics undoubtedly play a role in sleep disorders, it's essential to recognize that they are multifactorial, influenced by genetic, environmental, and lifestyle factors. Seeking professional evaluation and guidance is critical to managing these disorders and mitigating their impact on one's life.

5

The Science of Dreams

Dreams have long held a profound fascination for humanity. They are the enigmatic narratives that unfold within the theatre of our sleeping minds. In this realm, the boundaries of reality blur and imagination reign supreme. From dreams' vivid, surreal landscapes to their emotional impact, dreams have been a subject of intrigue, inspiration, and interpretation for centuries. In this chapter, we embark on a journey into the captivating world of dreams, guided by the light of scientific inquiry.

The Universal Language of Dreams

Dreams are a universal phenomenon experienced by people of all ages, cultures, and backgrounds. Whether they unfold as fleeting fragments or epic sagas, dreams are integral to the human experience. However, despite their ubiquity, studying dreams remains a complex and multifaceted.

Throughout human history, dreams have been attributed with significance and symbolism. Ancient civilizations sought meaning in dreams, viewing them as messages from the divine or glimpses into the future. Sigmund Freud, the pioneering psychologist, delved into the depths of the human psyche, introducing the concept of the unconscious mind and the interpretation of dreams as expressions of hidden desires and conflicts.

The Neurobiology of Dreaming

As our understanding of the brain and consciousness has advanced, so has our exploration of the science of dreams. Modern neuroscience has uncovered the intricate neural processes that underlie the act of dreaming. Research has revealed that dreaming is not confined to a single stage of sleep but occurs throughout various sleep cycles, most notably during Rapid Eye Movement (REM) sleep.

During REM sleep, the brain is highly active, and the eyes dart rapidly beneath closed lids—an apt description of the acronym. Dreams often take centre stage within this state, accompanied by increased brain activity in regions associated with emotions, memories, and vivid sensory experiences.

Dreams as a Window into the Mind

The science of dreams seeks to decode the cryptic language of the sleeping mind. It explores questions that have intrigued scientists, psychologists, and philosophers alike. What purposes do dreams serve, if any? Are they merely random brain activity, or do they hold deeper meanings? Can dreams provide insights into our emotions, fears, and unresolved conflicts?

Research has uncovered fascinating facets of dreaming, such as lucid dreaming, where individuals become aware of their dream state and, in some cases, gain control over the dream narrative. Additionally, studies have shown that dreams can influence mood, creativity, and problem-solving abilities.

The Therapeutic Potential of Dream Analysis

Dream analysis, a cornerstone of psychotherapy, offers a therapeutic approach to understanding the inner workings of the human psyche. Therapists use dreams to explore a patient's emotions, conflicts, and subconscious thoughts. By examining dream content and patterns, individuals can gain insight into their fears, desires, and unresolved issues, paving the way for personal growth and healing.

A Journey into the Dreaming Mind

In this chapter, we embark on a journey into dreams guided by scientific inquiry, neurological exploration, and psychological insight. We will explore the various stages of sleep and the role of dreams within them, shedding light on the neural processes that give rise to our nightly narratives. We will delve into the theories surrounding the purpose and significance of dreams and examine how dream analysis can be a valuable tool for self-discovery and emotional well-being.

As we navigate the landscapes of dreams, we invite you to join us in unravelling the mysteries of the sleeping mind. From the fantastical realms of dreamscapes to the inner recesses of the unconscious, we will seek to understand the profound impact of dreams on our waking lives and their role in shaping our understanding of ourselves.

The Nature of Dreams

Dreams, those ephemeral narratives that unfold within the confines of our slumbering minds, have fascinated and mystified us for millennia. As we delve into the intricate nature of dreams, we embark on a journey that transcends the boundaries of reality, exploring their purpose, the science behind them, and the theories that seek to decipher their cryptic messages.

The Enigmatic Realm of Dreams

Dreams, often shrouded in surrealism and ambiguity, constitute a natural yet enigmatic aspect of the human experience. They transport us to otherworldly landscapes, reunite us with long-lost loved ones, and evoke emotions ranging from joy to terror. Whether fleeting fragments or epic sagas, dreams serve as windows into the hidden corners of our consciousness.

Understanding Dreams and Their Purpose

Theories on the Function of Dreams

Throughout history, scholars and thinkers have proposed various theories about the purpose of dreams. While none provide a definitive answer, they offer intriguing insights:

1. **Psychoanalytic Theory (Sigmund Freud):** Freud posited that dreams serve as a portal to the unconscious mind, allowing us to explore repressed desires, fears, and unresolved conflicts. According to his theory, dream analysis can unveil the latent content concealed within dream symbols.

2. **Problem-Solving Theory (Carl Jung):** Jung believed dreams solve personal dilemmas and conflicts. He suggested that dreams draw upon the collective unconscious, providing guidance and insights for addressing life's challenges.

3. **Memory Consolidation Theory:** Some scientists propose that dreams play a role in consolidating and organizing memories. During sleep, the brain processes and stores information gathered throughout the day, possibly by creating dream narratives.

4. **Threat Simulation Theory:** Evolutionary psychologists propose that dreams may serve as simulations of threatening scenarios, allowing the dreamer to rehearse potential dangers and develop strategies for survival.

5. **Emotion Regulation Theory:** This theory suggests that dreams help regulate emotions. By experiencing intense emotions in the safe realm of dreams, individuals may become better equipped to manage similar emotions in waking life.

Dream States and Stages

Dreams are not uniform; they manifest during different sleep stages, each with distinct characteristics:

1. **REM Sleep Dreams:** Rapid Eye Movement (REM) sleep is often associated with vivid, emotionally charged dreams. During this stage, brain activity surges, and the eyes rush beneath closed eyelids. REM dreams are more likely to be remembered and can feature complex narratives.

2. **Non-REM Sleep Dreams:** Although less intense, dreams can occur during non-REM sleep. These dreams are often shorter, less vivid, and less emotionally charged than those in REM sleep.

Theories on Dream Interpretation

Deciphering dream content, known as dream interpretation, has been a subject of interest and debate for centuries. Various schools of thought have emerged, offering diverse approaches to understanding dreams. Some of the prominent theories on dream interpretation include:

1. Freudian Dream Analysis

Sigmund Freud, the father of psychoanalysis, believed that dreams were the "royal road to the unconscious." He proposed that dreams consist of two components: the manifest content (the dream as it appears) and the latent content (the hidden, symbolic meaning). Freud's approach involved delving beneath the surface of the dream to reveal the unconscious desires, fears and conflicts that it symbolically represented.

2. Jungian Dream Analysis

Carl Jung, a contemporary of Freud, expanded on dream analysis by introducing the concept of the collective unconscious. He suggested that dreams tap into a universal reservoir of shared symbols and archetypes. In Jungian analysis, dreams are seen as messages from the deeper self, offering guidance and insights into the dreamer's personal development.

3. Cognitive Dream Analysis

Cognitive psychology approaches dream analysis from a more rational perspective. Cognitive theorists propose that dreams are a product of the mind's attempt to process and organize information. Dream content may reflect the dreamer's mental processes, emotions, and thought patterns. This approach emphasizes the role of the dreamer's mind in constructing dream narratives.

4. Activation-Synthesis Theory

The activation-synthesis theory proposed by J. Allan Hobson and Robert McCarley suggests that dreams result from random neural activity during REM sleep. According to this theory, the brain attempts to make sense of these random signals by creating a narrative, leading to the experience of dreaming. In this view, dream content lacks inherent meaning and is a byproduct of neural processes.

5. Contemporary Approaches

Modern dream analysis incorporates elements of neuroscience, psychology, and cultural context. Some therapists and researchers focus on the emotional and psychological significance of dream symbols within the individual's life, while others explore the cultural and societal influences that shape dream content.

The Multifaceted Language of Dreams

Dreams continue to captivate and challenge our understanding. They are a canvas upon which the mind paints its most vivid and mysterious compositions. Whether viewed through the lens of Freudian symbolism, Jungian

archetypes, cognitive processing, or neurological randomness, dreams offer a multifaceted language that invites interpretation, exploration, and self-discovery.

Dreams are more than just fleeting images and emotions; they are the products of a complex interplay between consciousness and the unconscious mind. They serve as a mirror reflecting our innermost thoughts, desires, and fears while also occasionally offering glimpses into the collective human experience.

The Art of Dream Exploration

Dream interpretation is not a one-size-fits-all endeavour. It is an art that combines scientific knowledge with individual introspection. Theories on dream interpretation offer diverse tools for understanding the symbolic language of dreams, but they do not provide definitive answers. Instead, they invite us to embark on a personal journey of exploration.

In this chapter, we will navigate the intricate landscapes of dream analysis, exploring the theories, methods, and insights that have shaped our understanding of dreams throughout history. From Freudian psychoanalysis to contemporary approaches that blend psychology and neuroscience, we will uncover the richness of dream interpretation.

The study of dreams invites us to transcend the boundaries of wakefulness and venture into the realms of imagination and symbolism. It is a journey that extends beyond the realm of science and delves into the depths of the human psyche. As we explore the nature of dreams, we aim to unravel the mysteries concealed within their narratives, unlocking the potential for self-discovery, personal growth, and a deeper connection to the hidden recesses of our minds.

Lucid Dreaming and Sleep Paralysis

Lucid dreaming and sleep paralysis are two extraordinary phenomena that occur within sleep. Both offer unique and often surreal experiences, but they are distinct in their nature and impact. Further, we venture into the captivating world of lucid dreaming and the enigmatic territory of sleep paralysis, uncovering techniques for experiencing lucid dreams and strategies for dealing with sleep paralysis.

Lucid Dreaming: Unlocking the Dreamer's Realm

Lucid dreaming is when the dreamer becomes aware that they are dreaming while still immersed in the dream. This heightened awareness allows individuals to exert some degree of control over the dream narrative, creating a bridge between the conscious and subconscious mind. Lucid dreams can be vivid, exhilarating, and sometimes transformative experiences.

Techniques for Experiencing Lucid Dreams

1. Reality Testing:

Reality testing involves periodically questioning whether you are in a dream or awake daily. This habit can carry over into your dreams, where you may perform a reality check. You may realise you are dreaming if you find something unusual or contradictory within the dream.

2. Keep a Dream Journal:

Maintaining a dream journal is a valuable practice for anyone interested in lucid dreaming. Record your dreams as soon as you wake up, paying attention to recurring themes, characters, and settings. Over time, this can help you recognize patterns in your dreams and increase your chances of becoming lucid.

3. Mnemonic Induction of Lucid Dreams (MILD):

MILD is a technique developed by Dr. Stephen LaBerge, a pioneer in lucid dream research. It involves setting the intention to have a lucid dream and repeating a specific phrase or affirmation as you fall asleep, such as "I will realize I'm dreaming." The idea is to prime your subconscious mind for clarity.

4. Wake-Induced Lucid Dreams (WILD):

WILD is a technique that involves transitioning directly from wakefulness into a lucid dream state. It requires a state of relaxation and focus as you enter the dream consciously. This technique often requires sleep paralysis (which we will discuss later).

5. Wake-Back-to-Bed (WBTB):

WBTB involves waking up at night and staying awake for a short period (e.g., 20-30 minutes) before returning to sleep. This disrupts your normal sleep cycle and increases the likelihood of entering a dream while maintaining awareness.

The Benefits and Wonders of Lucid Dreaming

Lucid dreaming offers a wide range of benefits and experiences:

1. **Creative Exploration:** Lucid dreams provide a canvas for creative expression, allowing you to explore limitless worlds and scenarios.

2. **Overcoming Nightmares:** For some, lucid dreaming can be a tool for confronting and transforming nightmares into more positive or neutral experiences.

3. **Personal Growth:** Lucid dreaming can serve as a platform for self-discovery, problem-solving, and gaining insights into the subconscious mind.

4. **Enhanced Control:** Experienced lucid dreamers can actively shape their dream environments, engage in adventures, or even practice real-world skills within the dream state.

Sleep Paralysis: When Dreams Turn Haunting

In stark contrast to the freedom of lucid dreaming, sleep paralysis is an eerie phenomenon that occurs when an individual becomes temporarily paralyzed while transitioning between wakefulness and sleep or vice versa. During sleep paralysis, individuals may experience vivid and often frightening hallucinations. Intense fear or dread can accompany the inability to move or speak during this state.

Dealing with Sleep Paralysis

1. Stay Calm:

While it can be distressing, it's essential to remember that sleep paralysis is a natural phenomenon and typically temporary. Remind yourself that you are experiencing a sleep-related event.

2. Focus on Breathing:

If you are in a sleep paralysis episode, concentrate on regulating your breath. Slow, deep breaths can help ease feelings of panic.

3. Avoid Struggling:

Attempting to move or speak during sleep paralysis can lead to frustration and heightened anxiety. Instead, try remaining still and patient, knowing the episode will pass.

4. Visualize Positive Images:

Some individuals have reported that focusing on positive or calming mental images during sleep paralysis can help alleviate fear and discomfort.

5. Improve Sleep Hygiene:

Addressing underlying sleep issues, such as insomnia or sleep deprivation, can reduce the frequency of sleep paralysis episodes.

The Science Behind Sleep Paralysis

Sleep paralysis is thought to occur when the body briefly experiences a disruption in the sleep-wake cycle. During REM sleep, the brain typically signals the muscles to remain in temporary paralysis, preventing us from physically acting out our dreams. In sleep paralysis, this muscle atonia persists briefly, causing individuals to feel immobilized even as they regain consciousness.

The Intersection of Lucid Dreaming and Sleep Paralysis

Lucid dreaming and sleep paralysis share an intriguing intersection. Sleep paralysis often occurs when an individual becomes aware of their surroundings while their body remains in a state of muscle atonia. This can create a unique opportunity for those experienced in lucid dreaming to transition from sleep paralysis into a lucid dream state.

Technique for Transitioning from Sleep Paralysis to Lucid Dreaming:

1. During a sleep paralysis episode, focus on maintaining a calm and relaxed mind.

2. Visualize yourself entering a dream landscape. Imagine yourself floating or gently transitioning into a dream scenario.

3. As your mind becomes more immersed in the dream imagery, you may find yourself fully lucid within the dream.

This technique requires practice and familiarity with both sleep paralysis and lucid dreaming. It can offer a fascinating bridge between these two unusual states of consciousness.

Navigating the Borders of Sleep

Lucid dreaming and sleep paralysis represent sleep's intriguing and sometimes mysterious facets. While lucid dreaming allows us to explore the boundless realms of the mind, sleep paralysis presents an eerie threshold between wakefulness and slumber. Both phenomena remind us that the realm of sleep is far more complex, fascinating, and enigmatic than we often perceive.

Through techniques and understanding, we can embrace the wonders of lucid dreaming and navigate the eerie terrain of sleep paralysis. These experiences challenge our understanding of consciousness, offering windows into the depths of the mind and the boundaries of human perception.

The Profound Potential of Lucid Dreaming

Lucid dreaming is not merely an intriguing phenomenon; it can be a transformative and enlightening journey for those who explore its depths. The capacity to consciously navigate one's dreams opens doors to a realm where imagination knows no bounds. Here are some of the profound potentials of lucid dreaming:

1. Creative Exploration:

Lucid dreams are an artist's canvas, where creativity knows no limits. In this state, individuals can conjure up breathtaking landscapes, interact with intriguing characters, and explore fantastical realms. It's an opportunity to unleash the full spectrum of human imagination.

2. Emotional Healing:

For those grappling with past traumas or unresolved emotions, lucid dreaming can offer a safe space for emotional processing and healing. Dreamers can confront their fears, engage in cathartic experiences, and gain insights into their dynamic landscapes.

3. Problem Solving:

Lucid dreaming can be an invaluable tool for problem-solving. Individuals have reported finding solutions to real-world challenges within the landscape of their dreams. The dream state allows for creative brainstorming and experimentation, unburdened by the limitations of the waking world.

4. Personal Growth:

Exploring the depths of the subconscious mind in a lucid dream can lead to profound personal growth. Dreamers can confront their fears, address unresolved conflicts, and better understand their inner selves.

5. Spiritual Exploration:

Some individuals use lucid dreaming as a means of spiritual exploration. They may seek encounters with higher beings, explore expanded consciousness states, or engage in metaphysical experiences that challenge their understanding of reality.

The Intricate Tapestry of Sleep Paralysis

On the other side of the sleep spectrum lies sleep paralysis, a phenomenon that has sparked tales of the supernatural and haunted legends throughout history. However, it is essential to recognize that sleep paralysis, while unsettling, is a natural occurrence with scientific explanations.

1. Scientific Understanding:

Sleep paralysis is rooted in the intricate mechanisms of the sleep-wake cycle. During rapid eye movement (REM) sleep, the brain actively dreams while simultaneously inhibiting physical muscle movements through muscle atonia. In sleep paralysis, this muscle atonia lingers briefly as the individual transitions between sleep stages, causing the sensation of immobility.

2. Cultural Interpretations:

Across cultures, sleep paralysis has been interpreted in various ways. It is associated with supernatural entities like ghosts or demons in some societies. These cultural interpretations have given rise to accounts of "nightmares" or "hag-riding" experiences. Such interpretations can heighten the anxiety and fear experienced during sleep paralysis episodes.

3. Coping Strategies:

Dealing with sleep paralysis requires a combination of understanding and coping strategies. By recognizing it as a natural phenomenon, individuals can mitigate its fear. Practising relaxation techniques, maintaining good sleep hygiene, and addressing underlying sleep disorders can reduce the frequency of sleep paralysis episodes.

The Unique Intersection: Lucid Dreaming within Sleep Paralysis

The intersection of lucid dreaming and sleep paralysis is a captivating area of study and practice for those seeking to explore consciousness's boundaries. It highlights the plasticity and adaptability of the human mind even within states of transition between wakefulness and sleep.

This unique intersection offers an opportunity for dreamers to navigate the challenging landscape of sleep paralysis consciously. By maintaining a calm and focused state of mind during an episode, individuals may transition seamlessly from the unsettling sensation of immobility into the immersive world of lucid dreams.

Imagine the potential: turning a moment of fear and vulnerability into a doorway to boundless creativity and exploration. While mastering this transition can be challenging and requires practice, it showcases the incredible adaptability of the human mind even when it teeters on the edge of sleep.

Lucid dreaming and sleep paralysis represent two contrasting but equally fascinating aspects of the sleep experience. One invites us to explore the limitless landscapes of our imagination and consciousness, while the other challenges us to navigate the mysterious territory between wakefulness and slumber.

By delving into lucid dreaming practices and understanding the science behind sleep paralysis, we can embrace the full spectrum of our experiences during sleep. These phenomena remind us that the realm of sleep is not merely a passive state but a dynamic and vibrant landscape where the boundaries of reality and imagination blur, allowing us to expand our understanding of the human mind and consciousness.

6

Sleep and Mental Health

The intricate dance between sleep and mental health is a subject of growing fascination and concern in our modern world. While sleep has long been recognized as a fundamental pillar of overall well-being, the depth of its impact on mental health is only beginning to be fully understood. In this chapter, we embark on a journey to explore the profound connection between sleep and mental health, recognizing that our slumber's quality can shape our minds' landscape.

The Sleep-Mind Nexus

The relationship between sleep and mental health is complex and bidirectional, where each influences and interplays with the other. Sleep disturbances can lead to mental health challenges, and conversely, mental health disorders can disrupt our ability to obtain restorative sleep. This intricate interdependence underscores the significance of recognizing sleep as an essential component of mental wellness.

Sleep and Emotional Equilibrium

One of the most striking aspects of the sleep-mind connection is its impact on emotional equilibrium. Sleep is a time of emotional processing and regulation, where the brain sifts through the day's experiences, categorizing memories and emotions. Adequate and restful sleep consolidates positive emotional memories while tempering the intensity of negative ones.

Conversely, sleep deprivation can lead to heightened emotional reactivity, irritability, and increased vulnerability to stress. Chronic sleep problems may contribute to the development of mood disorders such as depression and anxiety, creating a cycle where sleep disturbances exacerbate emotional difficulties and vice versa.

The Role of Sleep in Cognitive Function

Sleep is critical in cognitive functions such as memory consolidation, problem-solving, and decision-making. During the various stages of sleep, the brain processes and organizes information acquired during waking hours. Adequate sleep fosters clear thinking, efficient learning, and enhanced creativity.

Conversely, sleep deprivation impairs cognitive function, leading to memory, attention, and executive functioning deficits. Chronic sleep deficits may contribute to cognitive decline and increase the risk of neurodegenerative disorders like Alzheimer's disease.

Sleep Disorders and Mental Health

Sleep disorders such as insomnia, sleep apnea, and restless leg syndrome can disrupt the delicate balance between sleep and mental health. These conditions not only lead to daytime fatigue and impair cognitive function but also contribute to mood disorders and exacerbate pre-existing mental health conditions.

Understanding the bidirectional relationship between sleep disorders and mental health is crucial. Treating sleep disorders can alleviate symptoms of mood and anxiety disorders while addressing underlying mental health issues can lead to improvements in sleep quality.

The Impact of Stress and Trauma

Stress and trauma are potent disruptors of both sleep and mental health. The body's stress response, characterized by the release of cortisol, can interfere with the ability to fall asleep and stay asleep. Chronic stress and exposure to traumatic events can lead to conditions like post-traumatic stress disorder (PTSD) and insomnia.

Moreover, sleep disturbances can perpetuate the effects of stress and trauma, hindering the process of emotional recovery and exacerbating symptoms of mental health disorders.

The Influence of Lifestyle Factors

Lifestyle factors such as irregular sleep schedules, excessive screen time, and poor sleep hygiene can compound the challenges faced by those with mental health disorders. These factors disrupt the circadian rhythm, making it difficult to establish consistent sleep patterns.

This chapter will delve into the intricate connections between sleep and mental health. We will explore the role of sleep in emotional regulation, cognitive function, and overall well-being. We will examine the impact of sleep disorders, stress, and trauma on mental health, recognizing the importance of early intervention and holistic approaches to treatment.

As we navigate the terrain of sleep and mental health, we will uncover practical strategies for improving sleep quality and promoting mental wellness. Our exploration serves as a reminder that sleep is not a passive state but a dynamic force that can shape the landscape of our minds, influencing our emotional equilibrium, cognitive abilities, and overall mental health.

Sleep and Emotional Well-being

Sleep, that nightly voyage into dreams, is far more than a biological necessity. It is an intricate and dynamic process that holds the power to shape our emotional well-being. In exploring the profound connection between sleep and emotional health, we uncover the intricate dance between the two and discover how managing stress and anxiety through better sleep can lead to a happier, more balanced life.

The Bidirectional Relationship Between Sleep and Mental Health

The relationship between sleep and emotional well-being is reciprocal, where each influences and amplifies the other. Understanding this complex interplay is essential to appreciating the role of sleep in maintaining a stable dynamic equilibrium.

1. Sleep Impacts Emotions:

A night of disrupted sleep can lead to increased emotional reactivity, heightened stress levels, and a greater vulnerability to negative emotions. The brain's ability to regulate emotions becomes compromised when sleep is insufficient or of poor quality.

2. Emotional State Affects Sleep:

Conversely, our emotional state significantly influences our ability to obtain restorative sleep. Anxiety, depression, and stress can lead to insomnia and fragmented sleep patterns. This creates a cycle where emotional difficulties disrupt sleep, exacerbating emotional challenges.

3. Mood Disorders and Sleep:

Mood disorders, such as depression and bipolar disorder, often manifest with disrupted sleep patterns. Insomnia is a common symptom of depression, while individuals with bipolar disorder may experience manic episodes that disrupt sleep, followed by depressive periods with excessive sleepiness.

Managing Stress and Anxiety Through Better Sleep

Recognizing the bidirectional relationship between sleep and emotional well-being underscores the importance of nurturing healthy sleep habits to manage stress and anxiety effectively. Here are some practical strategies to achieve this balance:

1. Prioritize Sleep Hygiene:

Establishing a sleep-conducive environment and routine is crucial. Maintain a consistent sleep schedule, create a comfortable sleeping space, and avoid stimulating activities before bedtime. These practices signal to your body that it's time to wind down.

2. Mindfulness and Relaxation Techniques:

Mindfulness meditation, deep breathing exercises, and progressive muscle relaxation can help reduce stress and anxiety. Engaging in these practices before bedtime can promote relaxation and improve sleep quality.

3. Limit Screen Time:

Exposure to screens before bed can disrupt melatonin production, a hormone that regulates sleep. Reduce screen time, especially exposure to the blue light emitted by phones, tablets, and computers, in the hours leading up to bedtime.

4. Manage Worry and Rumination:

Excessive worry and rumination are common contributors to insomnia and poor sleep. Practice techniques to manage these thoughts, such as journaling, setting aside designated "worry time" during the day, and cognitive-behavioural therapy (CBT).

5. Regular Exercise:

Engaging in regular physical activity can promote better sleep and alleviate symptoms of anxiety and depression. Aim for at least 30 minutes of moderate exercise most days of the week, but avoid vigorous exercise close to bedtime.

6. Limit Caffeine and Alcohol:

Both caffeine and alcohol can disrupt sleep patterns. Limit their consumption, especially in the hours before bedtime, to ensure better sleep quality.

The Ripple Effect on Emotional Well-being

Recognizing the profound impact of sleep on emotional well-being reveals the potential for a ripple effect. By nurturing healthy sleep habits and managing stress and anxiety through better sleep, individuals can experience a transformation in their overall emotional state.

The path to emotional well-being may begin with something as simple as a good night's sleep. By prioritizing rest, practising relaxation techniques, and addressing the bidirectional relationship between sleep and emotions, we can create a positive cycle where improved sleep leads to enhanced emotional well-being and vice versa.

In the intricate dance between sleep and emotional health, we find a pathway to resilience, dynamic equilibrium, and a happier, more balanced life. We can unlock the potential for lasting well-being and greater emotional harmony through these practices and a deeper understanding of the connection between sleep and emotions.

The Power of Emotional Regulation Through Sleep

Emotional regulation is one of the most remarkable aspects of the sleep-emotion connection. Sleep acts as a natural regulator of emotions, helping individuals process and cope with the challenges they face during the day. Here's how it works:

1. Emotional Memory Processing:

During the various stages of sleep, the brain processes emotional memories, categorizing and integrating them into existing knowledge. This process allows individuals to gain perspective on their emotional experiences and reduce the emotional intensity associated with distressing memories.

2. Stress Reduction:

A whole night's sleep helps regulate the body's stress response. Cortisol, the stress hormone, follows a natural circadian rhythm, peaking in the morning and gradually decreasing throughout the day. However, chronic sleep deprivation disrupts this rhythm, leading to heightened cortisol levels and increased vulnerability to stress.

3. Dream Therapy:

Dreams affect emotional regulation, particularly during REM (Rapid Eye Movement) sleep. Dreaming provides a safe space for processing emotions, exploring unresolved conflicts, and rehearsing problem-solving scenarios. Dreams can serve as expressive therapy, helping individuals understand their feelings.

The Importance of Seeking Balance

Balancing sleep and emotional well-being requires a holistic approach encompassing sleep hygiene and self-care. Acknowledging the interconnectedness of these two aspects of well-being allows individuals to cultivate a more resilient and emotionally balanced life.

1. Self-Compassion:

Cultivating self-compassion is a fundamental component of emotional well-being. Recognize that occasional sleep disturbances are a part of life. Be kind to yourself when sleep doesn't go as planned, and avoid self-criticism or worry about its potential impact.

2. Professional Support:

If sleep problems persist or are accompanied by severe emotional challenges, seeking professional help is essential. Mental health professionals can provide tailored strategies and therapies to address sleep disturbances and emotional difficulties.

3. Lifestyle Integration:

Incorporate emotional self-care practices into your daily routine. This may include mindfulness meditation, journaling, hobbies, or spending time with loved ones. These practices can help alleviate stress and promote emotional resilience.

4. Balanced Nutrition:

A well-balanced diet can contribute to better sleep quality and emotional well-being. Avoid excessive caffeine and sugar intake, as they can disrupt sleep patterns and emotional stability. Instead, prioritize a diet rich in whole foods and nutrients that support brain health.

The Path to Emotional Harmony

Navigating the complex relationship between sleep and emotional well-being can profoundly transform one's life. Recognizing the bidirectional influence of these factors empowers individuals to take charge of their emotional health by prioritizing sleep and adopting healthy, dynamic self-care practices.

As we journey through the chapters of this book, we will delve deeper into the intricate connections between sleep, mental health, and emotional well-being. Individuals can unlock the potential for greater emotional harmony, resilience, and well-being by understanding and implementing strategies to nurture these connections.

Embracing sleep as a vital ally in the pursuit of emotional well-being reveals the profound power of a good night's rest. In the sleep-emotion dance, we find the rhythm of dynamic equilibrium, allowing us to navigate life's challenges with grace, self-compassion, and a peaceful heart.

Sleep and Cognitive Function

The relationship between sleep and cognitive function is profound, touching on memory, creativity, and problem-solving. In this exploration, we delve into how sleep impacts these critical facets of our cognitive abilities and unveil strategies for enhancing cognitive function through the power of sleep.

The Remarkable Impact of Sleep on Memory

Sleep is a time of memory consolidation and optimization. While you slumber, your brain actively processes and organizes the information gathered during waking hours. This memory-related phenomenon occurs during different stages of sleep, with each phase contributing to specific memory functions.

1. Short-Term Memory:

During the lighter stages of non-REM (Rapid Eye Movement) sleep, your brain processes and consolidates short-term memories acquired throughout the day. This phase is crucial for retaining information temporarily, allowing you to recall details from recent experiences.

2. Long-Term Memory:

The deep, slow-wave stages of non-REM sleep play a pivotal role in transferring information from short-term to long-term memory storage. This process, known as memory consolidation, strengthens neural connections and enhances your ability to recall information for the long haul.

3. Emotional Memory:

REM sleep, often associated with vivid dreaming, is instrumental in processing emotional memories. It helps us make sense of emotionally charged experiences, allowing us to gain insight and find emotional closure.

4. Spatial Memory:

Sleep is also linked to spatial memory, which involves recalling locations and spatial relationships. Adequate sleep fosters a deeper understanding of spatial environments and can improve navigation skills.

The Creative Potential of Sleep

Creativity thrives in the fertile grounds of sleep. It's common to wake up with fresh ideas, innovative solutions, or newfound inspiration after a good night's rest. Here's how sleep cultivates creativity:

1. Associative Thinking:

During REM sleep, the brain engages in associative thinking, making unexpected connections between unrelated ideas. This creative process, often evident in dreams, can lead to innovative insights and problem-solving.

2. Problem-Solving in Dreams:

The phenomenon of "dreaming solutions" is well-documented. Individuals have reported dreaming about challenging problems and waking up with a newfound understanding of how to solve them. This illustrates the power of sleep in facilitating creative problem-solving.

3. Enhanced Divergent Thinking:

Divergent thinking, a key component of creativity, involves generating many ideas from a single starting point. Adequate sleep has been shown to enhance divergent thinking, allowing individuals to explore a broader range of creative possibilities.

The Role of Sleep in Problem-Solving

Sleep can be a valuable ally when tackling complex problems and making decisions. Here's how sleep contributes to effective problem-solving:

1. Unconscious Processing:

During sleep, the brain works on unresolved problems and complex information. It sifts through data, processes it, and extracts insights, often leading to "aha" moments upon waking.

2. Insight Formation:

Sleep fosters the formation of insights, those sudden and profound realizations that bring clarity to challenging situations. The " incubation " process during sleep allows the brain to reorganize information and uncover novel solutions.

3. Decision-Making Clarity:

Adequate sleep improves decision-making by enhancing cognitive function and clarity. Well-rested individuals are better equipped to evaluate options, weigh pros and cons, and make sound decisions.

Strategies for Improving Cognitive Function Through Sleep

Harnessing the full potential of sleep for cognitive function involves adopting strategies prioritising sleep quality and quantity. Here are some practical approaches:

1. Prioritize Sleep Hygiene:

Establish a consistent sleep schedule and create a conducive sleep environment. Keep your bedroom calm, dark, and quiet. Limit exposure to screens before bedtime, as the blue light emitted can disrupt melatonin production.

2. Sleep Duration:

As experts recommend, aim for 7-9 hours of sleep per night. This duration allows for adequate time in each sleep stage, facilitating memory consolidation, creative thinking, and problem-solving.

3. Strategic Naps:

Short naps, often called power naps, can boost cognitive function and creativity. A 20-30-minute nap can provide a mental refresh without the grogginess of longer naps.

4. Mindfulness Meditation:

Engage in mindfulness meditation practices, which can improve sleep quality and enhance cognitive function. These practices promote relaxation, reduce stress, and contribute to overall well-being.

5. Regular Exercise:

Incorporate regular physical activity into your routine. Exercise not only promotes better sleep but also enhances cognitive function and creativity.

6. Avoid Sleep Disruptors:

Limit the consumption of caffeine and alcohol, especially in the hours leading up to bedtime. These substances can disrupt sleep patterns and impair cognitive function.

The Cognitive Symphony of Sleep

In the symphony of cognitive function, sleep plays a vital role as the conductor, orchestrating memory consolidation, nurturing creativity, and facilitating problem-solving. By understanding the profound impact of sleep on cognitive abilities and adopting strategies for optimizing sleep, individuals can unlock their mental potential, leading to enhanced memory, creativity, and problem-solving skills.

As we continue to explore the fascinating relationship between sleep and cognitive function, we gain insight into the intricate workings of the mind and uncover the remarkable benefits that sleep bestows upon our cognitive abilities. Sleep is an indispensable ally in the quest for optimal cognitive function, guiding us toward the zenith of mental insight and creativity.

The Cognitive Renaissance: Nurturing Your Brain through Sleep

To further appreciate the transformative potential of sleep on cognitive function, let's explore real-world scenarios where sleep can make a tangible difference:

1. Learning and Education:

For students and learners of all ages, sleep is an invaluable ally in pursuing knowledge. Adequate sleep enhances memory consolidation, making retaining and recalling information easier. Whether studying for exams, acquiring new skills, or delving into a new subject, prioritizing sleep can significantly boost your learning capabilities.

2. Problem-Solving in the Workplace:

Solving complex problems and making well-informed decisions is a prized asset in the professional realm. Sleep contributes to cognitive clarity and insight formation, allowing individuals to tackle intricate challenges easily. Well-rested employees often exhibit greater creativity and problem-solving skills, enhancing productivity and innovation.

3. Creativity in the Arts:

Creatives, from artists and writers to musicians and designers, often rely on their imaginative prowess to produce compelling work. Sleep's role in nurturing creativity is particularly evident in artistic endeavours. By fostering divergent thinking and facilitating associative connections, sleep can inspire artists to produce their most innovative and meaningful creations.

4. Mental Resilience:

In our fast-paced and demanding world, maintaining mental resilience is essential. Sleep contributes to emotional stability, stress reduction, and the ability to adapt to challenges. A well-rested mind is better equipped to face adversity with clarity and composure.

Cultivating a Sleep-Enhanced Lifestyle

The strategies for enhancing cognitive function through sleep extend beyond sleep hygiene practices. They encompass a holistic approach to lifestyle choices and habits that prioritize restorative slumber:

1. Mindful Consumption:

Monitor your caffeine and alcohol intake, especially in the hours preceding bedtime. These substances can interfere with sleep quality and disrupt the sleep cycle.

2. Stress Management:

Use stress-reduction techniques such as meditation, yoga, or deep breathing exercises. These practices can calm the mind and improve sleep quality.

3. Balanced Diet:

Nutrition plays a significant role in sleep quality. Maintain a balanced diet rich in whole foods, and consider eating lighter meals in the evening to avoid discomfort during sleep.

4. Regular Physical Activity:

Incorporate regular exercise into your routine, but avoid vigorous exercise close to bedtime. Exercise can promote better sleep and enhance overall cognitive function.

5. Consistent Sleep Schedule:

Establish and maintain a consistent sleep schedule, even on weekends. Consistency reinforces your body's internal clock, making it easier to fall asleep and wake up at the desired times.

6. Technology Moderation:

Limit exposure to screens before bedtime, as the blue light emitted by devices can suppress melatonin production and disrupt sleep patterns.

The Path to Cognitive Excellence

Embracing the remarkable connection between sleep and cognitive function and applying these strategies to your life, you embark on a journey toward mental excellence. With improved memory, creativity, and problem-solving skills, you can navigate the complexities of daily life with greater ease and confidence.

In exploring the cognitive symphony of sleep, we have uncovered the profound influence that sleep holds over memory, creativity, and problem-solving. Sleep emerges not only as a physiological necessity but also as a catalyst for cognitive brilliance. By nurturing this relationship and allowing sleep to work its magic, individuals can elevate their cognitive abilities to new heights, reaching for the peaks of mental acuity and creative insight.

As we journey through the chapters of this book, we continue to unveil the multifaceted wonders of sleep and its impact on our well-being. Each exploration gives us a deeper understanding of how sleep can empower us to lead more vibrant, creative, and intellectually fulfilling lives.

7

Sleep and Physical Health

In the intricate tapestry of our lives, the significance of sleep extends far beyond the realm of mere rest. It weaves through the fabric of our physical health, influencing every system, organ, and function within our bodies. As we embark on this journey into the profound interplay between sleep and physical well-being, we uncover sleep's essential role in nurturing and sustaining our bodies.

The Inextricable Bond: Sleep and Physical Health

The connection between sleep and physical health is both profound and intricate. It's a relationship where each facet of well-being relies on the other, forming an inseparable bond. At the heart of this bond lies the recognition that sleep is not just a passive state but a dynamic and essential force that supports and sustains our bodies.

1. Restorative Power:

At its core, sleep is a time of restoration and repair. While we slumber, our bodies undergo intricate processes promoting healing, growth, and vitality. During this rest period, the body addresses the wear and tear of daily life, rejuvenating tissues and replenishing energy reserves.

2. Immune Vigilance:

Sleep is an unsung hero of the immune system. It enhances the production of immune cells and proteins that defend the body against infections and illnesses. When sleep is compromised, the immune system weakens, making us more susceptible to infections and hampering our recovery.

3. Hormonal Harmony:

The endocrine system, responsible for regulating hormones, relies on sleep for balance. Adequate sleep supports the regulation of hormones that control appetite, metabolism, stress response, and growth. Sleep disruptions can lead to hormonal imbalances with far-reaching effects on physical health.

4. Cardiovascular Well-being:

Sleep plays a pivotal role in cardiovascular health. It contributes to maintaining healthy blood pressure, heart rate, and overall cardiovascular function. Chronic sleep deprivation has been linked to an increased risk of heart disease, stroke, and other cardiovascular conditions.

5. Metabolic Resilience:

The metabolic processes that govern blood sugar regulation and weight management are intricately linked to sleep. Sleep deficiency can disrupt these processes, increasing the risk of metabolic disorders such as diabetes and obesity.

Sleep as the Guardian of Physical Health

Sleep is a guardian of physical health, defending the body against stress, illness, and daily wear and tear. It is a powerful ally that supports the body's natural capacity to heal, grow, and thrive. Yet, in our fast-paced world, the importance of sleep is often overlooked or sacrificed at the altar of productivity and convenience.

The Disruptive Forces: Sleep Disorders

While sleep is a powerful force for physical health, sleep disorders can disrupt this delicate equilibrium. Conditions such as sleep apnea, insomnia, and restless leg syndrome can undermine the body's ability to achieve restorative sleep, leading to a cascade of health challenges.

1. Sleep Apnea:

Obstructive sleep apnea, characterized by pauses in breathing during sleep, is associated with an increased risk of cardiovascular disease, hypertension, and cognitive impairment. Its disruptive nature robs individuals of the rejuvenating effects of restorative sleep.

2. Insomnia:

Chronic insomnia, characterized by difficulty falling or staying asleep, can have far-reaching consequences for physical health. It is linked to an increased risk of mental health disorders, cardiovascular disease, and compromised immune function.

3. Restless Leg Syndrome:

This condition, characterized by uncomfortable sensations in the legs and an irresistible urge to move them, can lead to chronic sleep disruption. It often results in daytime fatigue and an increased risk of mood disorders.

The Holistic Approach to Physical Health

Our exploration into the relationship between sleep and physical health underscores the importance of adopting a holistic approach to well-being. Recognizing sleep as a cornerstone of physical health empowers individuals to take proactive steps to nurture their bodies.

1. Prioritizing Sleep Hygiene:

A consistent sleep schedule and a sleep-conducive environment are essential to sleep hygiene. These practices ensure that the body receives the restorative sleep it needs.

2. Managing Stress:

Stress management techniques, such as meditation, yoga, and relaxation exercises, can alleviate the burden of stress on physical health and improve sleep quality.

3. Seeking Treatment for Sleep Disorders:

For those grappling with sleep disorders, seeking treatment is crucial. Consultation with healthcare professionals can lead to tailored therapies and interventions that address the underlying causes of sleep disturbances.

4. Nutrition and Physical Activity:

A balanced diet and regular physical activity improve sleep quality and overall physical health. Avoiding excessive caffeine and alcohol consumption, especially before bedtime, is also essential.

The Uncharted Territories of Physical Health

As we delve deeper into the chapters of this book, we uncover the uncharted territories where sleep holds sway over physical health. We examine the intricate processes during sleep, the disruptive forces of sleep disorders, and the holistic approaches that empower individuals to protect and enhance their physical well-being.

In this chapter, we embark on a journey to explore the vast landscapes where sleep and physical health converge. We recognize sleep not only as a passive state but as a dynamic and essential force that nurtures, sustains, and defends our bodies. Together, we unravel the profound interplay between sleep and physical well-being, offering insights and strategies for cultivating a healthier, more resilient body.

Sleep and Physical Health

In the hustle and bustle of our modern lives, sleep is often relegated to the back burner, sacrificed for productivity, entertainment, or simply a packed schedule. Yet, the importance of sleep for physical health cannot be overstated. It's not merely a luxury or a passive state but an essential component of our well-being. In this exploration, we delve into the profound role of sleep in maintaining physical health and unveil the stark effects of sleep deprivation on the body.

The Role of Sleep in Maintaining Physical Health

A Nightly Restoration Process

Think of sleep as a nightly restoration process for your body. When you drift off into slumber, your body doesn't just shut down; it gets to work. While you rest, your body is busy repairing tissues, synthesizing proteins, and bolstering the immune system.

Immune System Support

One of the critical roles of sleep is supporting the immune system. During the deep stages of sleep, your body ramps up the production of immune cells and proteins. These immune warriors stand ready to defend your body against infections, viruses, and harmful pathogens. A good night's sleep equips your immune system with the ammunition it needs to keep you healthy.

Hormonal Harmony

The endocrine system, responsible for regulating hormones, relies on sleep to maintain balance. Sleep helps regulate hormones that control appetite, metabolism, stress response, and growth. When sleep is disrupted, hormones can go awry, leading to potential health issues.

Cardiovascular Well-being

Sleep also plays a pivotal role in cardiovascular health. It contributes to the maintenance of healthy blood pressure and heart rate. Chronically disturbed sleep can lead to an increased risk of heart disease, stroke, and other cardiovascular conditions.

Metabolic Resilience

Sleep is a crucial player in metabolic processes, such as blood sugar regulation and weight management. Sleep deficiency can disrupt these processes, potentially leading to metabolic disorders like diabetes and obesity.

Emotional Stability

Your emotional well-being is intimately connected to your physical health, and sleep serves as a stabilizing force. Adequate sleep reduces the risk of mood disorders and fosters emotional resilience. On the flip side, sleep deprivation can exacerbate stress, anxiety, and depression.

Effects of Sleep Deprivation on the Body

The Underestimated Consequences

Now that we've glimpsed the remarkable roles that sleep plays in maintaining physical health, it's time to confront the harsh reality of sleep deprivation and its consequences. The effects of sleep deprivation are often underestimated, but they have far-reaching implications for our bodies.

Cognitive Impairment

Sleep deprivation can wreak havoc on cognitive function. It impairs memory, attention, and problem-solving abilities. You might find concentrating, making decisions, or recalling information harder when you sleep too little.

Mood Swings

Emotional instability often accompanies sleep deprivation. You may become irritable, moody, or prone to mood swings. Simple tasks can feel overwhelming, and stress levels tend to soar.

Weakened Immunity

Remember how sleep supports the immune system? Well, sleep deprivation does the opposite. It weakens your body's defences, making you more susceptible to infections, colds, and other illnesses. You're essentially disarming your immune warriors by skimping on sleep.

Weight Gain

Sleep and metabolism go hand in hand. Sleep deprivation disrupts the hormones that regulate appetite, often leading to increased cravings for sugary and high-calorie foods. This can, in turn, contribute to weight gain and obesity over time.

Increased Risk of Chronic Conditions

The consequences of chronic sleep deprivation are particularly dire. It's associated with an increased risk of severe health conditions like heart disease, diabetes, and hypertension. The longer you skimp on sleep, the higher the stakes become.

Reduced Physical Performance

Sleep deprivation can significantly hinder performance for those who engage in physical activities or sports. It impairs coordination, reaction time, and muscle recovery. Athletes often prioritize sleep as an essential component of their training regimen.

A Wake-Up Call: The Need for Quality Sleep

The implications are clear: sleep is not a negotiable aspect of our lives but an essential one. It's not something we can trade for extra hours of work or entertainment without consequences. Neglecting sleep comes at a price, and that price is our physical health.

Actionable Advice for Quality Sleep

Prioritize Sleep Hygiene

Establish a consistent sleep schedule and create a sleep-conducive environment. Keep your bedroom calm, dark, and quiet. Limit exposure to screens before bedtime, as the blue light emitted can disrupt melatonin production.

Get Your Hours In

As experts recommend, aim for 7-9 hours of sleep per night. This duration allows for adequate time in each sleep stage, facilitating memory consolidation, immune support, and overall physical well-being.

Mindful Consumption

Monitor your caffeine and alcohol intake, especially in the hours leading up to bedtime. These substances can interfere with sleep quality and disrupt the sleep cycle.

Stress Management

Use stress-reduction techniques such as meditation, yoga, or deep breathing exercises. These practices can calm the mind and improve sleep quality.

Regular Physical Activity

Incorporate regular exercise into your routine, but avoid vigorous exercise close to bedtime. Exercise promotes better sleep and enhances overall physical health.

A Vital Partnership: Sleep and Physical Health

In conclusion, the partnership between sleep and physical health is not a matter of choice but a necessity. It's a dynamic relationship where sleep actively contributes to our well-being, and its absence takes a toll on our bodies. It's time we acknowledge the pivotal role of sleep in maintaining physical health and take proactive steps to prioritize our sleep. By doing so, we invest in our physical well-being, allowing our bodies to thrive, heal, and flourish as they are meant to do. Sleep, after all, is not just a passive state; it's a vital force that sustains the essence of our physical existence.

Navigating the Real-World Challenges

Understanding the intricate dance between sleep and physical health is only part of the equation. In the real world, we face numerous challenges and lifestyle factors that can impact our ability to get quality sleep. Let's delve deeper into these challenges and explore strategies to overcome them:

1. The 24/7 Society:

Our modern, interconnected world operates on a 24/7 basis. The advent of technology has brought about the constant availability of information and entertainment, blurring the boundaries between day and night. Many individuals find it challenging to disconnect and wind down in the evening, leading to sleep disturbances.

Actionable Strategy: Establish digital boundaries. Create a digital curfew by turning off screens at least an hour before bedtime. Use this time for relaxation and winding down with activities like reading, gentle stretching, or practising mindfulness.

2. Work and Stress:

Work-related stress is a significant contributor to sleep problems. High-pressure jobs, long working hours, and constant communication through emails and messages can lead to heightened stress levels and difficulty unwinding.

Actionable Strategy: Implement stress management techniques. Whether it's through meditation, progressive muscle relaxation, or deep breathing exercises, finding ways to manage and alleviate work-related stress is crucial for a good night's sleep.

3. Shift Work:

Shift work, which involves irregular work hours outside the typical 9-to-5 schedule, can wreak havoc on the body's natural sleep-wake rhythm. It can lead to sleep disorders, including shift work disorder, which manifests as insomnia and excessive daytime sleepiness.

Actionable Strategy: Create a sleep-friendly shift work routine. Ensure your sleep environment is conducive to rest by making it as dark and quiet as possible. Consider using blackout curtains and white noise machines to create a sleep-conducive atmosphere.

4. Travel and Jet Lag:

Travelling across time zones can disrupt your internal body clock, resulting in the dreaded jet lag. The misalignment between your body's circadian rhythm and the local time can lead to sleep difficulties and discomfort.

Actionable Strategy: Gradually adjust your sleep schedule. Before your trip, gradually shift your bedtime and wake time closer to your destination's time zone.

Upon arrival, spend time outdoors in natural light to help reset your internal clock.

5. Medications and Medical Conditions:

Certain medications and medical conditions can interfere with sleep. For example, stimulants, antidepressants, and medicines for high blood pressure can disrupt sleep patterns. Chronic pain conditions or respiratory disorders like sleep apnea can also lead to sleep disturbances.

Actionable Strategy: Consult with healthcare professionals. If you suspect that medications or medical conditions are affecting your sleep, seek guidance from healthcare providers. They can adjust medications or provide treatments to improve sleep quality.

6. Lifestyle Choices:

Daily habits, such as excessive caffeine or alcohol consumption, irregular mealtimes, and lack of physical activity, can negatively impact sleep. Poor dietary choices and a sedentary lifestyle can contribute to sleep problems and affect overall physical health.

Actionable Strategy: Adopt a balanced lifestyle. Pay attention to your dietary choices, exercise regularly, and monitor caffeine and alcohol intake, especially during bedtime. A balanced lifestyle can improve both sleep quality and physical health.

Embracing the Journey to Better Sleep and Physical Health

The journey to better sleep and enhanced physical health has its challenges. It requires a mindful approach, understanding the unique factors that influence our sleep, and a commitment to prioritising sleep.

Recognizing that sleep is not a passive state but an active contributor to our physical well-being empowers us to take charge of our health. By embracing a holistic perspective that encompasses sleep hygiene, stress management, and lifestyle choices, we can unlock the full potential of sleep in nurturing our bodies.

The following chapters will delve into the multifaceted relationship between sleep and physical health. We will explore the specific aspects of sleep, from its impact on the immune system to its role in maintaining cardiovascular well-being. Armed with knowledge and actionable strategies, we can navigate the complexities of our modern world while prioritizing sleep as an essential cornerstone of our physical health. The journey may have challenges, but the rewards are immeasurable—a healthier, more vibrant you.

Sleep and Chronic Illness

In our fast-paced world, the importance of sleep often takes a backseat to the demands of daily life. We might sacrifice a few hours of sleep to meet work deadlines, binge-watch our favourite shows, or catch up on social media. However, what many fail to realize is that chronic sleep deprivation can have severe consequences for our long-term health, contributing to the development and exacerbation of chronic illnesses like diabetes, heart disease, and obesity.

The Link Between Sleep and Chronic Illness

Diabetes: A Disrupted Metabolism

The connection between sleep and diabetes is intricate and multifaceted. Sleep deprivation can disrupt the body's ability to regulate blood sugar levels, leading to insulin resistance and an increased risk of type 2 diabetes. When we don't get enough sleep, our bodies produce less insulin and are less efficient at removing glucose from the bloodstream, contributing to elevated blood sugar levels.

Moreover, sleep deprivation affects our appetite-regulating hormones, increasing cravings for sugary and high-calorie foods. This, in turn, can contribute to weight gain and obesity, which are significant risk factors for diabetes.

Heart Disease: The Silent Threat

Sleep and heart health are intimately linked. Chronic sleep deprivation can elevate the risk of heart disease in several ways. Firstly, it can lead to elevated blood pressure, a well-established risk factor for cardiovascular problems. When we don't get enough restorative sleep, our blood pressure remains elevated for extended periods, placing strain on the heart and blood vessels.

Secondly, sleep deficiency can lead to the accumulation of plaque in the arteries, a condition known as atherosclerosis. This buildup restricts blood flow, increasing the risk of heart attacks and strokes. Sleep apnea, a sleep disorder characterized by pauses in breathing during sleep, is closely associated with heart disease. It can lead to irregular heart rhythms and further stress the cardiovascular system.

Obesity: The Vicious Cycle

The relationship between sleep and obesity is a complex one. Sleep deprivation disrupts the balance of hunger-regulating hormones, increasing appetite and cravings for unhealthy foods. This can lead to overeating and weight gain. Simultaneously, obesity can exacerbate sleep problems, such as sleep apnea and insomnia, creating a vicious cycle.

Lack of sleep also impairs our ability to make healthy food choices and engage in regular physical activity. Fatigue and low energy levels often deter individuals from exercise, further contributing to obesity and related health issues.

Lifestyle Changes to Improve Sleep and Reduce the Risk of Illness

Prioritize Sleep Hygiene

1. **Establish a Consistent Sleep Schedule:** Go to bed and wake up simultaneously every day, even on weekends. This helps regulate your body's internal clock.

2. **Create a Sleep-Conducive Environment:** Make your bedroom a haven for sleep. Keep it calm, dark, and quiet. Invest in a comfortable mattress and pillows.

3. **Limit Screen Time Before Bed:** The blue light emitted by phones, tablets, and computers can interfere with the production of melatonin, a hormone that regulates sleep. Aim to avoid screens at least an hour before bedtime.

Manage Stress

1. **Practice Relaxation Techniques:** Engage in stress-reduction activities such as meditation, deep breathing exercises, or progressive muscle relaxation.

2. **Establish Boundaries:** Set boundaries between work and personal life. Avoid checking work emails or engaging in work-related tasks before bedtime.

Regular Physical Activity

1. **Incorporate Exercise:** Aim for at least 30 minutes of moderate-intensity exercise most days of the week. Regular physical activity can improve sleep quality and overall health.

2. **Timing Matters:** While exercise is beneficial, avoid vigorous workouts close to bedtime, as they can be stimulating and interfere with sleep.

Diet and Nutrition

1. **Watch Your Diet:** Be mindful of what you eat, especially in the hours leading up to bedtime. Avoid heavy or spicy meals, as they can cause discomfort during sleep.

2. **Limit Caffeine and Alcohol:** Reduce caffeine and alcohol intake, especially in the afternoon and evening. These substances can disrupt sleep patterns.

Technology Moderation

1. **Digital Curfew:** Establish a digital curfew by turning off screens at least an hour before bedtime. Use this time for relaxation and enjoy activities like reading or listening to soothing music.

Seek Professional Help

1. **Consult a Healthcare Provider:** If you're struggling with chronic sleep problems or suspect a sleep disorder, seek guidance from a healthcare professional. They can diagnose and treat underlying issues like sleep apnea or insomnia.

Weight Management

1. **Maintain a Healthy Weight:** If you're overweight or obese, work on gradual weight loss through a balanced diet and regular exercise. Weight loss can improve sleep quality and reduce the risk of obesity-related health issues.

The Path to Wellness

In conclusion, the relationship between sleep and chronic illness is undeniable. Sleep deprivation can disrupt metabolism, elevate blood pressure, and contribute to the development of conditions like diabetes, heart disease, and obesity. However, the path to wellness is equally clear. By prioritizing sleep, adopting healthy lifestyle choices, and seeking professional guidance when needed, we can break the cycle of sleep deficiency and reduce the risk of chronic illness.

Understanding the vital connection between sleep and health is the first step. Implementing actionable strategies and embracing a holistic approach to well-being is the path to a healthier, more vibrant life. Sleep is not just a luxury; it's an essential component of our overall health, and by nurturing it, we invest in a brighter and healthier future.

Embracing a Healthier Future: Sleep as Your Ally

As we continue to explore the profound relationship between sleep and chronic illness, it's crucial to recognize that the journey to better health is multifaceted. While improving sleep quality plays a pivotal role, it's just one piece of the puzzle. Embracing a holistic approach to wellness encompasses various aspects of life that influence both sleep and overall health.

Mental Health and Sleep

Mental health is closely intertwined with both sleep and chronic illness. Conditions such as depression and anxiety can lead to sleep disturbances, while sleep deprivation can exacerbate mental health challenges. It's a bidirectional relationship that underscores the importance of addressing mental well-being as part of the journey to better sleep and physical health.

Stress Reduction

Stress is a common factor that can disrupt sleep patterns and contribute to chronic illnesses. Chronic stress triggers the release of stress hormones, which can lead to insomnia and other sleep problems. Conversely, poor sleep can increase stress levels, creating a vicious cycle.

Actionable Strategy: Implement stress reduction techniques such as mindfulness meditation, yoga, or progressive muscle relaxation. These practices can help calm the mind and improve sleep quality.

Mental Health Support

If you're experiencing mental health challenges, seek professional help. Therapy, counselling, and support groups can provide valuable tools and resources to manage and overcome mental health conditions. Addressing these issues can positively impact both sleep and overall well-being.

Social Connections and Sleep

Our social interactions and relationships also play a role in sleep and chronic illness. Loneliness and social isolation have been linked to sleep disturbances, while strong social connections can provide emotional support and improve sleep quality.

Prioritize Relationships

Cultivating meaningful relationships with friends and family can provide a sense of belonging and support. Spending time with loved ones, engaging in social activities, and maintaining a support network can positively influence mental health and sleep.

Limit Social Media

While staying connected through social media is valuable, excessive screen time, especially before bedtime, can interfere with sleep. Create boundaries by disconnecting from screens at least an hour before sleep to improve sleep hygiene.

Environmental Influences and Sleep

The physical environment in which you live can significantly impact sleep quality and chronic illness risk.

Light Exposure

Exposure to natural light during the day helps regulate your body's internal clock and sleep-wake cycle. However, excessive light exposure at night, especially from electronic screens, can disrupt melatonin production and hinder sleep.

Actionable Strategy: Spend time outdoors during the day, and ensure your sleep environment is as dark as possible at night. Consider using blackout curtains and minimizing electronic devices in the bedroom.

Noise Reduction

A quiet sleep environment is essential for quality rest. Noise disturbances from traffic, neighbours, or other sources can lead to fragmented sleep and increased stress levels.

Actionable Strategy: Use white noise machines or earplugs to mask disruptive sounds and create a peaceful sleep atmosphere.

A Balanced Approach to Nutrition

Nutrition is a cornerstone of health, and dietary choices can influence both sleep and the risk of chronic illness.

Balanced Diet

A balanced diet rich in whole foods, fruits, vegetables, lean proteins, and healthy fats supports overall health and can improve sleep quality. Avoid excessive consumption of processed or sugary foods, especially in the hours before bedtime.

Actionable Strategy: Pay attention to your diet and aim for nutritious meals with essential vitamins and minerals. Avoid heavy or spicy meals close to bedtime to prevent discomfort during sleep.

Medications and Medical Conditions

Certain medications and medical conditions can interfere with sleep and contribute to chronic illness risk. It's essential to work closely with healthcare professionals to manage these factors.

Medication Management

If you're taking medications that affect sleep, consult with your healthcare provider. They may adjust dosages or recommend alternative treatments to minimize sleep disruption.

Chronic Illness Management

If you have a chronic illness, following your treatment plan and managing the condition effectively is crucial. This can include medications, lifestyle changes, and regular medical check-ups to monitor your health.

The Road Ahead: Empowering Your Wellness Journey

The path to better sleep and reduced risk of chronic illness is a dynamic journey encompassing various facets of life. It's about recognizing the interplay between sleep, mental health, social connections, the environment, nutrition, and medical factors. By embracing a holistic approach to well-being and implementing actionable strategies in these areas, you empower yourself to take control of your health.

Remember that small, sustainable changes can yield significant results over time. Prioritizing sleep, nurturing your mental health, fostering social connections, creating a sleep-conducive environment, making nutritious food choices, and managing medications and medical conditions all contribute to your overall well-being.

As you embark on this journey, celebrate each step forward and acknowledge that your efforts are investments in a healthier, more vibrant future. Sleep is not a passive state; it's a powerful ally in your quest for long-lasting wellness. With each night of restorative slumber, you move closer to a healthier, more fulfilled life where sleep and well-being walk hand in hand.

8

Sleep Solutions and Strategies

In our quest to unravel the mysteries of sleep and explore its profound impact on our lives, we have journeyed through the intricate terrain of restful slumber. We've delved into the science behind sleep, unravelled its connection to physical and mental health, and unearthed the hidden world of dreams. As we venture into this chapter, we stand at the threshold of a new realm—Sleep Solutions and Strategies.

Sleep, that invaluable companion to our daily existence, can sometimes prove elusive. Whether it's the ceaseless chatter of a busy mind, the persistent pull of digital devices, or the trials of a demanding schedule, sleep can slip through our fingers like grains of sand. But worry not, for within these pages, we will equip you with a treasure trove of insights, techniques, and practical wisdom to reclaim the restorative power of sleep.

The Complex Landscape of Sleep Solutions

Sleep is not a one-size-fits-all proposition. The solutions and strategies that help one person sleep like a baby may not be the panacea for another. That's why we embark on this chapter with a deep understanding of the complexity of sleep and a recognition that the path to restful nights is as diverse as the individuals seeking it.

The Sleep-Deprived Society

In our modern world, the pace of life often seems relentless. The demands of work, family, and personal pursuits can leave us feeling perpetually sleep-deprived. The consequences of this chronic sleep deficiency are far-reaching, affecting our physical health, emotional well-being, and cognitive function.

Unlocking the Secrets of Sleep

As we journey through this chapter, we will unlock the secrets of sleep and reveal the strategies that can lead to better sleep hygiene and sleep quality. We will explore the importance of a consistent sleep schedule, the benefits of creating a sleep-conducive environment, and the role of relaxation techniques in preparing the mind and body for rest.

The Multifaceted Nature of Sleep Solutions

The solutions to our sleep woes are multifaceted, encompassing a broad spectrum of approaches that cater to different needs and preferences. Within these pages, you will encounter a rich tapestry of techniques and strategies, each offering a unique path to restful slumber.

Sleep Hygiene: The Foundation of Quality Sleep

We begin with the cornerstone of sleep solutions—sleep hygiene. This encompasses practices and habits that form the bedrock of healthy sleep patterns. Sleep hygiene lays the foundation for restful nights, from establishing a consistent sleep schedule to creating a sleep-conducive environment.

Relaxation and Mindfulness: Calming the Restless Mind

Finding solace for the mind is often the key to a peaceful night's sleep in a world of distractions and anxieties. We will explore relaxation and mindfulness techniques to help calm the restless mind, banishing the worries that can keep us tossing and turning.

Sleep Aids and Supplements: Tools for Troubled Sleepers

For those grappling with chronic sleep problems, sleep aids and supplements can offer valuable support. We will delve into the world of sleep aids, exploring their benefits, potential risks, and how to use them judiciously.

Technology and Sleep: Navigating the Digital Age

In an age defined by technology, our devices can be our allies or adversaries when it comes to sleep. We will guide you through the digital landscape, offering insights into how to harness technology to improve sleep quality and when to unplug for a peaceful night's rest.

Sleep Disorders: Seeking Professional Help

For those facing persistent and debilitating sleep problems, the chapter will guide them on when to seek professional help. We will explore common sleep disorders, their symptoms, and the available treatment options to help you regain sleep control.

Empowering Your Sleep Journey

As we embark on this chapter, remember that the solutions and strategies you encounter are not mandates but tools for your toolbox. Each individual's journey to restful sleep is a personal and unique one. What works best for you may require some experimentation and adaptation. The key is to embark on this journey with an open heart and a willingness to explore the possibilities.

Whether seeking a good night's sleep to enhance your physical health, nurture your emotional well-being, or awaken each day with a sharper mind, this chapter holds the answers you seek. The landscape of sleep solutions is vast and ever-evolving, and by delving into its depths, you empower yourself to take control of your sleep and embrace the vitality it brings to your life.

Sleep Aids and Medications

Sleep, that elusive realm of rest and rejuvenation, often dances out of reach for many of us. The search for solutions intensifies when tossing and turning becomes the nightly ritual. Among the arsenal of strategies to combat insomnia and sleep disorders, sleep aids and medications stand as potent allies. In this exploration, we delve into sleep aids and medications, understanding their role, potential benefits, and the considerations accompanying their use.

The Quest for Quality Sleep

The quest for quality sleep can be a relentless pursuit for those who grapple with sleepless nights. Sleep, a fundamental pillar of well-being, is critical for physical, mental, and emotional health. Chronic sleep deprivation can take a toll on our lives, leading to fatigue, irritability, reduced cognitive function, and a heightened risk of health issues.

Sleep Deprivation: A Global Challenge

The pervasive problem of sleep deprivation is a global challenge. The demands of modern life, including work schedules, digital distractions, and the pressures of daily existence, often leave us yearning for a good night's sleep. When sleep becomes an elusive commodity, many individuals turn to sleep aids and medications for respite.

The Role of Sleep Aids and Medications

Sleep aids, and medications can offer a lifeline to those in the throes of sleeplessness. They are designed to help individuals fall asleep faster, stay asleep longer, and experience a more profound, refreshing slumber. However, it's crucial to recognize that sleep aids are not one-size-fits-all solutions. Their effectiveness varies depending on the underlying causes of sleep disturbances and individual differences in response.

Types of Sleep Aids and Medications

The landscape of sleep aids and medications is diverse, encompassing various categories and formulations:

1. Over-the-counter (OTC) Sleep Aids: These are available without a prescription and typically contain antihistamines, such as diphenhydramine or doxylamine. They are designed to induce drowsiness and can be helpful for occasional sleep problems.

2. Prescription Sleep Medications: These are available only with a prescription from a healthcare provider. They include medications like zolpidem (Ambien), eszopiclone (Lunesta), and zaleplon (Sonata). These medications target specific receptors in the brain to promote sleep.

3. Melatonin Supplements: Melatonin is a hormone naturally produced by the body that helps regulate sleep-wake cycles. Melatonin supplements are available over-the-counter and can be helpful for individuals with circadian rhythm disruptions or jet lag.

4. Herbal and Natural Remedies: Some individuals use herbal supplements like valerian root, chamomile, or CBD products for sleep support. The efficacy of these remedies can vary, and somebody should consider their safety.

When to Consider Sleep Aids and Medications

The decision to use sleep aids and medications should be made thoughtfully and in consultation with a healthcare provider. Doctors should be consulted under the following circumstances:

1. Short-Term Sleep Problems:

Occasional bouts of insomnia due to stress, jet lag, or other transient factors may benefit from short-term use of sleep aids.

2. Chronic Sleep Disorders:

Individuals diagnosed with chronic sleep disorders like insomnia, sleep apnea, or restless leg syndrome may be prescribed specific medications as part of their treatment plan.

3. Lifestyle Disruptions:

Shift workers, frequent travellers, and individuals with irregular schedules may use sleep aids to help regulate their sleep patterns.

4. Medical Conditions:

Certain medical conditions, such as chronic pain, anxiety, or depression, can contribute to sleep disturbances. In some cases, medications prescribed to manage these conditions may also improve sleep.

Considerations and Precautions

While sleep aids and medications can be valuable tools in the pursuit of better sleep, they come with considerations and precautions:

1. Potential Side Effects:

Sleep medications can cause side effects, including dizziness, drowsiness, headache, and impaired coordination. It's essential to be aware of these potential effects, especially when driving or operating heavy machinery.

2. Risk of Dependency:

Some prescription sleep medications have the potential for dependency or addiction if not used as directed. It's crucial to follow healthcare provider recommendations closely and use them only for the prescribed duration.

3. Tolerance and Reduced Efficacy:

Over time, the body may tolerate the effects of certain sleep medications, leading to reduced efficacy. This can necessitate dosage adjustments or changes in treatment.

4. Interaction with Other Medications:

Sleep medications can interact with other medicines, supplements, or alcohol. It's vital to inform healthcare providers of all drugs and substances being used to prevent adverse interactions.

5. Cognitive Impairment:

Certain sleep aids can lead to cognitive impairment the following day, affecting memory, attention, and decision-making. It's essential to allow sufficient time for rest after taking these medications.

Lifestyle and Behavioral Approaches

In tandem with sleep aids and medications, lifestyle and behavioural approaches play a crucial role in improving sleep quality. These approaches include:

1. Sleep Hygiene: Establishing good sleep hygiene practices, such as maintaining a consistent sleep schedule, creating a comfortable sleep environment, and limiting screen exposure before bedtime.

2. Relaxation Techniques: Incorporating relaxation techniques like deep breathing, progressive muscle relaxation, or meditation into the bedtime routine to calm the mind and body.

Cognitive Behavioral Therapy for Insomnia (CBT-I): A structured therapeutic approach that helps individuals identify and address the thoughts and behaviours contributing to sleep problems.

Healthy Lifestyle Choices: Adopting a balanced diet, regular physical activity, and stress management practices that promote overall well-being and improve sleep quality.

The Decision-Making Process

Ultimately, the decision to use sleep aids and medications should be collaborative between individuals and their healthcare providers. It involves a comprehensive evaluation of sleep patterns, medical history, and potential underlying causes of sleep disturbances.

While sleep aids and medications can relieve those in need, they are most effective when integrated into a holistic approach to sleep improvement. Individuals can optimize their chances of achieving restful, restorative sleep by combining medication with lifestyle and behavioural changes.

In pursuing sleep solutions, it's essential to remain open to the diversity of approaches available. What works best for one person may not be the answer for another. The journey to restful slumber is a unique and individual one, and by exploring the multifaceted landscape of sleep aids and medications, individuals can empower themselves to take control of their sleep and awaken each day refreshed and revitalized.

Overview of Common Sleep Aids: Navigating the Path to Restful Slumber

Sleep is a fundamental aspect of our lives, essential for maintaining physical and mental health. Yet, many find the quest for a peaceful night's sleep elusive. Sleep aids, a diverse category of remedies and medications, offer a range of options to help individuals overcome sleep disturbances and achieve restorative rest. In this exploration, we embark on a journey through the common sleep aids available, understanding their mechanisms, benefits, and considerations for use.

The Pervasive Problem of Sleeplessness

Chronic sleep deprivation is a pervasive problem in our modern world. Stress, lifestyle, medical conditions, and even digital distractions can disrupt our natural sleep patterns. When sleeplessness becomes a persistent challenge, searching for adequate sleep aids becomes increasingly essential.

The Consequences of Sleep Deprivation

The consequences of sleep deprivation are far-reaching, impacting not only our physical health but also our cognitive function, emotional well-being, and overall quality of life. Sleepless nights can lead to fatigue, irritability, decreased productivity, impaired memory, and an increased risk of chronic health conditions.

Common Sleep Aids: An Array of Options

The world of sleep aids is diverse, offering various options to address sleep disturbances and insomnia. These aids can broadly be categorized into several groups:

1. Over-the-counter (OTC) Sleep Aids:

OTC sleep aids are readily available without a prescription, making them accessible to individuals seeking relief from occasional sleep problems. They typically contain antihistamines such as diphenhydramine or doxylamine. These antihistamines induce drowsiness and can be effective for short-term use.

Benefits:

- Convenience: OTC sleep aids are available in most drugstores and do not require a prescription.

- Short-Term Relief: They can be helpful for individuals experiencing temporary sleep disruptions, such as travel-related jet lag or occasional insomnia.

Considerations:

- Tolerance: OTC sleep aids may become less effective as the body develops tolerance.

- Side Effects: They can cause side effects such as drowsiness, dry mouth, and dizziness.

- Potential Dependency: Long-term use can lead to dependency or the need for higher doses.

2. Melatonin Supplements:

Melatonin is a hormone naturally produced by the body to regulate the sleep-wake cycle. Melatonin supplements, available over-the-counter, are designed to help individuals with circadian rhythm disruptions or jet lag.

Benefits:

- Circadian Regulation: Melatonin supplements can help reset the internal body clock and improve sleep timing.

- Non-Habit Forming: Melatonin supplements are generally considered non-habit forming.

Considerations:

- Timing Matters: The timing of melatonin supplements is crucial for their effectiveness.

- Individual Response: The response to melatonin supplements varies among individuals.

4. Herbal and Natural Remedies:

Some individuals use herbal supplements like valerian root, chamomile, lavender, or CBD products to promote relaxation and sleep. These remedies are available over-the-counter.

Benefits:

- Natural Approach: Herbal remedies are perceived as natural and have fewer side effects.

- Relaxation: They can induce a sense of relaxation and calm.

Considerations:

- Efficacy Variability: The efficacy of herbal remedies can vary, and scientific evidence may be limited.

- Consultation: Individuals should consult a healthcare provider before using herbal remedies, especially if taking other medications.

Risks and Benefits of Medication for Sleep

The use of sleep medications offers both benefits and potential risks that individuals should carefully consider:

Benefits:

1. **Improved Sleep Onset:** Medications can help individuals fall asleep faster, reducing the time spent lying in bed.

2. **Extended Sleep Duration:** Some medications promote more prolonged periods of uninterrupted sleep, increasing overall sleep duration.

3. **Enhanced Sleep Quality:** Certain medications can improve sleep architecture, leading to deeper and more restorative sleep.

Risks:

1. **Dependency and Tolerance:** Long-term use of some sleep medications can lead to dependence and tolerance, requiring higher doses for the same effect.

2. **Side Effects:** Sleep medications can cause side effects, including drowsiness, dizziness, headache, gastrointestinal disturbances, and impaired coordination.

3. **Cognitive Impairment:** Some medications can lead to cognitive impairment the following day, affecting memory, attention, and decision-making.

4. **Interaction with Other Medications:** Sleep medications can interact with other medicines, supplements, or alcohol, potentially leading to adverse effects or reduced efficacy.

5. **Limited Long-Term Use:** Many sleep medications are intended for short-term use, and their long-term safety and efficacy are not well-established.

The Decision-Making Process

The decision to use sleep aids or medications should be made thoughtfully and in consultation with a healthcare provider. It involves a comprehensive evaluation of an individual's sleep patterns, medical history, and potential underlying causes of sleep disturbances.

While sleep aids and medications can relieve those in need, they are most effective when integrated into a holistic approach to sleep improvement. Individuals can optimize their chances of achieving restful, restorative sleep by combining medication with lifestyle and behavioural changes.

In pursuing sleep solutions, it's essential to remain open to the diversity of approaches available. What works best for one person may not be the answer for another. The journey to restful slumber is a unique and individual one, and by exploring the multifaceted landscape of sleep aids and medications, individuals can empower themselves to take control of their sleep and awaken each day refreshed and revitalized.

Natural Sleep Remedies

In the realm of sleep, the quest for restful nights often leads us to explore the healing power of nature. Natural sleep remedies, often rooted in centuries-old traditions and wisdom, offer a gentle and holistic approach to overcoming insomnia and sleep disturbances. In this exploration, we journey through natural sleep remedies, uncovering their mechanisms, benefits, and considerations for those seeking tranquil repose.

The Allure of Natural Sleep Remedies

In a world brimming with technology and the hustle and bustle of daily life, the allure of natural sleep remedies lies in their simplicity and connection to the natural world. These remedies draw upon herbs, plants, and relaxation techniques cherished for generations for their potential to induce peaceful slumber.

A Return to Natural Healing

Natural sleep remedies provide a compelling alternative to conventional medications for individuals seeking a more gentle and holistic approach to sleep. They often embrace the philosophy that the body has an innate ability to heal itself when provided with the right tools and conditions.

The Multifaceted World of Natural Sleep Remedies

Natural sleep remedies encompass a wide range of approaches, each with its unique mechanisms and benefits. These remedies have been categorized into several groups:

1. Herbal Sleep Aids:

Herbal remedies harness the power of specific plants and herbs traditionally used for their calming and soothing properties. Some commonly used herbs for sleep include:

Valerian Root: Valerian is known for its mild sedative effects and has been used for centuries to promote relaxation and sleep.

Chamomile: Chamomile is renowned for its soothing properties and can be brewed into a relaxing tea.

Lavender: Lavender essential oil or sachets can create a calming sleep environment.

Passionflower: Passionflower is believed to reduce anxiety and improve sleep quality.

Benefits:

- Natural Approach: Herbal remedies are derived from plants and are perceived as genuine and safe.

- Relaxation can induce relaxation and calmness, helping individuals unwind before bedtime.

Considerations:

- Variability: The efficacy of herbal remedies can vary among individuals, and scientific evidence may be limited.

- Consultation: Individuals should consult a healthcare provider, especially if taking other medications.

2. Aromatherapy:

Aromatherapy utilizes essential oils extracted from plants to create a soothing ambience. Essential oils like lavender, chamomile, and cedarwood can be diffused or applied topically to promote relaxation and sleep.

Benefits:

- Relaxing Atmosphere: Aromatherapy can transform your sleep environment into a tranquil sanctuary.

- Stress Reduction: The inhalation of calming scents can reduce stress and anxiety.

Considerations:

- Dilution: Essential oils should be diluted appropriately and used with care to prevent skin irritation.

- Individual Sensitivity: Some individuals may have sensitivities or allergies to specific essential oils.

3. Mindfulness and Relaxation Techniques:

Mindfulness practices, such as meditation, progressive muscle relaxation, and deep breathing exercises, are natural approaches that calm the mind and reduce stress.

Benefits:

- Stress Reduction: Mindfulness techniques can alleviate stress and anxiety, common contributors to sleep disturbances.

- Improved Sleep Quality: Consistent practice can lead to better sleep quality and an enhanced ability to manage sleep-related stress.

Considerations:

- Practice: Mastery of these techniques often requires consistent practice over time.

- Individual Response: The effectiveness of mindfulness techniques can vary among individuals.

4. Dietary Adjustments:

Diet plays a pivotal role in sleep quality. Certain foods and beverages can promote restful sleep, while others can disrupt it.

a. Foods Promoting Sleep:

Certain foods like bananas, almonds, turkey, and warm milk contain sleep-promoting nutrients like tryptophan and melatonin.

b. Herbal Teas:

Herbal teas like chamomile, valerian root, and passionflower can induce relaxation before bedtime.

Benefits:

- Nutritional Support: Consuming sleep-promoting foods and beverages can provide nutritional support for better sleep.

- Hydration: Herbal teas can contribute to hydration and relaxation.

Considerations:

- Timing: To avoid discomfort during sleep, foods and beverages should be consumed right.

- Dietary Sensitivities: Individuals with food allergies or sensitivities should choose remedies carefully.

Holistic Benefits and Considerations

Natural sleep remedies offer holistic benefits beyond inducing sleep. They can address the underlying factors contributing to sleep disturbances, such as stress, anxiety, and poor sleep hygiene. Additionally, they often provide a sense of empowerment, allowing individuals to participate in their sleep improvement journey actively.

Benefits of Natural Remedies:

1. **Gentle Approach:** Natural remedies are generally mild and have fewer side effects than medications.

2. **Stress Reduction:** Many natural remedies focus on reducing stress and anxiety, which can contribute to sleeplessness.

3. **Holistic Approach:** These remedies often address multiple aspects of well-being, promoting overall health.

4. **Empowerment:** Using natural remedies can empower individuals to take control of their sleep and explore self-care practices.

Considerations:

1. **Efficacy Variability:** The effectiveness of natural remedies can vary among individuals, and results may not be immediate.

2. **Consultation:** Individuals with underlying medical conditions or medications should consult a healthcare provider before using natural remedies.

3. **Consistency:** Some natural remedies, such as mindfulness, require consistent practice to yield significant benefits.

Crafting Your Sleep Sanctuary

The world of natural sleep remedies invites individuals to craft their sleep sanctuary—a space where the mind and body can unwind, relax, and embrace the refreshing embrace of sleep. Combining these remedies with good sleep hygiene practices, such as maintaining a consistent sleep schedule and creating a comfortable sleep environment, can enhance their effectiveness.

Natural sleep remedies offer a holistic and empowering path in pursuing restful slumber. By drawing from the healing power of nature, individuals can nurture their well-being, reduce stress, and rediscover the joy of serene sleep. Ultimately, the journey to tranquil repose is personal and unique, and natural sleep remedies provide a tapestry of options for individuals to explore as they unlock the secrets to restful nights.

9
The Future of Sleep Science

As we journey through the realms of slumber, exploring the intricacies of sleep and its profound impact on our lives, we find ourselves standing at the precipice of possibility. Chapter 9 ushers us into the fascinating world of "The Future of Sleep Science." Here, we venture beyond the boundaries of what we know today, peering into the ever-evolving landscape of sleep research and the exciting discoveries that await us.

The Enigma of Sleep

Sleep, that enigmatic state of being, has long captured the curiosity of scientists, philosophers, and dreamers alike. Its mysteries are woven into the fabric of our existence, touching every aspect of our physical, mental, and emotional well-being. Yet, despite centuries of inquiry, sleep remains one of human existence's most profound and enigmatic phenomena.

The Multifaceted Nature of Sleep

Throughout this journey, we've delved into the multifaceted nature of sleep, unravelling its diverse components—the sleep-wake cycle, circadian rhythms, sleep architecture, dreams, and the intricate web of factors that influence the quality of our rest. We've explored the science behind sleep disorders, the role of sleep in mental and physical health, and the array of strategies and remedies to enhance our sleep.

The Quest for Deeper Understanding

Our exploration has revealed that the world of sleep is not static but a dynamic and evolving field of study. Sleep scientists and researchers continue to push the boundaries of knowledge, peeling back the layers of complexity that shroud sleep's secrets. An insatiable curiosity drives them to understand this vital aspect of human existence's underlying mechanisms, functions, and potential.

Emerging Frontiers in Sleep Research

The future of sleep science promises to open new frontiers and explore uncharted territories. Researchers are poised to unveil discoveries that could transform how we understand and approach sleep. This chapter will journey through some of the most promising and exciting emerging frontiers in sleep research.

The Role of Technology

One of the most remarkable aspects of the future of sleep science is the role of technology. We live in an era of rapid advancements in digital tools, wearable devices, and neuroimaging techniques. These innovations have empowered scientists to delve deeper into the mysteries of the sleeping brain and the intricacies of our sleep patterns.

Wearable Sleep Monitoring Devices

Wearable devices with sensors that track heart rate, movement, and brain activity have provided individuals unprecedented insights into their sleep. These devices can potentially revolutionize our understanding of sleep patterns and disorders, empowering individuals to proactively optimise their sleep.

Neuroimaging and Sleep Research

Advancements in neuroimaging, such as functional magnetic resonance imaging (fMRI) and electroencephalography (EEG), offer scientists a window into the sleeping brain. These technologies enable researchers to observe brain activity during different sleep stages and explore the neural correlates of dreams, sleep disorders, and cognitive processes.

Personalized Sleep Medicine

A shift toward personalized sleep medicine marks the future of sleep science. Rather than adopting a one-size-fits-all approach to sleep disorders and disturbances, healthcare providers are increasingly tailoring treatments to individual needs.

Genomic Sleep Medicine

Genomic research is unveiling the genetic underpinnings of sleep disorders. Understanding an individual's genetic predisposition to certain sleep conditions can inform personalized treatment strategies and therapeutic interventions.

Precision Therapies

In the years to come, we can expect the development of precision therapies that target the specific mechanisms underlying sleep disorders. These therapies will aim to provide more effective and tailored solutions for individuals with diverse sleep challenges.

Exploring the Mind in Sleep

The future of sleep science will also venture deeper into exploring the dreaming mind. Dreams have long captivated our imagination, and emerging research is shedding light on the purpose and significance of these nightly journeys.

Dream Research and Mental Health

Researchers are investigating the relationship between dreams and mental health, exploring how dream content and patterns may provide insights into emotional well-being and the processing of traumatic experiences.

Lucid Dreaming and Consciousness

The phenomenon of lucid dreaming, where individuals are aware they are dreaming and may exert control over their dreams, continues to intrigue researchers. The study of lucid dreaming holds promises for understanding the nature of consciousness itself.

The Intersection of Sleep and Technology

The future of sleep science will increasingly intersect with the digital world. Technology will play a pivotal role in shaping the future of sleep improvement, from AI-driven sleep coaches to immersive sleep environments.

AI-Powered Sleep Solutions

Artificial intelligence and machine learning algorithms are harnessed to develop personalized sleep improvement plans. These AI-driven sleep coaches can analyze an individual's sleep data and provide tailored recommendations for better sleep.

Immersive Sleep Environments

Virtual reality (VR) and augmented reality (AR) technologies are being explored to create immersive sleep environments that enhance sleep quality and promote relaxation.

The Journey Ahead

As we embark on this chapter, we invite you to join us in peering into the future of sleep science, where possibilities are as limitless as the dreams that visit us each night. Together, we will explore cutting-edge research, technological innovations, and evolving paradigms that promise to deepen our understanding of sleep and enhance the quality of our lives.

In this chapter, we will delve into the exciting frontiers of sleep research, embrace the holistic approach to sleep, and unravel the intricate connections between sleep and our physical and mental well-being—the future of sleep science beckons. We are poised to answer its call.

Ongoing Research and Discoveries

The realm of sleep, often shrouded in darkness and mystery, is witnessing a profound transformation. In the world of sleep science, ongoing research and discoveries are shedding new light on the enigmatic nature of slumber. As we peer into the current studies and breakthroughs in sleep research, we unveil the exciting possibilities that await, promising a deeper understanding of sleep and its far-reaching implications for human health and well-being.

Current Studies and Breakthroughs in Sleep Research

1. The Brain in Sleep: Unveiling the Secrets of Dreams

One of the most captivating areas of ongoing research is the study of the sleeping brain. Neuroimaging techniques like functional magnetic resonance imaging (fMRI) and electroencephalography (EEG) have allowed researchers to peer into the brain's inner workings during different sleep stages. These technologies are enabling scientists to decode the neural patterns associated with dreams.

Recent breakthroughs in dream research have uncovered surprising connections between dream content and emotional processing. Studies suggest that dreams are crucial in emotional regulation and memory consolidation. They may serve as a nocturnal therapy session, helping individuals process and make sense of their waking experiences. Researchers are also delving into the neural correlates of lucid dreaming, a state where individuals are aware they are dreaming, offering insights into the nature of consciousness itself.

2. Genetics and Sleep Disorders: Unlocking the Genetic Code

The study of genetics is revolutionizing our understanding of sleep disorders. Researchers are identifying specific genes and genetic variations associated with sleep disturbances, such as insomnia, sleep apnea, and restless legs syndrome. This genetic insight paves the way for personalized treatments tailored to an individual's genetic profile.

Genomic sleep medicine is on the horizon, potentially revolutionising the diagnosis and treatment of sleep disorders. Genetic markers may help predict an individual's risk of developing sleep disorders and guide therapeutic interventions. Ongoing research is unravelling the intricate genetic tapestry of sleep, providing hope for more effective and targeted treatments.

3. Sleep and Mental Health: A Bidirectional Relationship

The intricate relationship between sleep and mental health remains a focal point of research. Current studies are shedding light on the bidirectional nature of this relationship. On one hand, sleep disturbances can contribute to the development and exacerbation of mental health conditions such as depression and anxiety. On the other hand, mental health challenges can lead to sleep disturbances.

Breakthroughs in this field elucidate the underlying mechanisms connecting sleep and mental health. For example, research has shown that sleep disturbances can disrupt the brain's emotional regulation circuits, contributing to mood disorders. Conversely, effective treatment of sleep disorders can lead to improvements in mental health.

4. Sleep Quality and Physical Health: A Holistic Approach

The intricate connections between sleep quality and physical health are a constant source of fascination for researchers. Ongoing studies uncover sleep's far-reaching impact on various facets of physical well-being, including cardiovascular health, metabolic function, and immune system resilience.

Recent discoveries highlight the importance of sleep quality, not just quantity, in maintaining physical health. Sleep fragmentation, characterized by frequent awakenings during the night, is emerging as a potential risk factor for health conditions such as hypertension and obesity. Understanding the role of sleep architecture and sleep continuity in physical health is a burgeoning area of research.

What the Future Holds for Understanding Sleep

As we peer into the future of sleep science, a tapestry of possibilities unfurls before us. These possibilities offer a more profound comprehension of sleep and the potential to transform how we approach sleep-related challenges and disorders.

1. Personalized Sleep Medicine: Tailoring Treatment to Individuals

The future of sleep medicine is increasingly personalized. Advances in genetic research and diagnostics are paving the way for tailored treatments that address the specific factors contributing to an individual's sleep disturbances. Personalized sleep medicine will encompass a holistic approach, addressing both the physiological and psychological aspects of sleep.

2. Precision Therapies for Sleep Disorders: Targeting Mechanisms

Emerging research is poised to uncover the precise mechanisms underlying sleep disorders. This understanding will enable the development of precision therapies that target the root causes of sleep disturbances. Rather than relying solely on symptomatic relief, these therapies will address the underlying issues, offering more effective and lasting solutions.

3. Sleep and Technology: The Digital Revolution

Technology is poised to play a pivotal role in the future of sleep science. Wearable devices with sophisticated sensors and AI algorithms offer individuals unprecedented insights into their sleep patterns. These devices empower individuals to take an active role in optimizing their sleep and provide valuable data for research.

Virtual reality (VR) and augmented reality (AR) technologies are being explored to create immersive sleep environments that enhance sleep quality and promote relaxation. AI-driven sleep coaches analyse vast datasets to provide personalized recommendations for improving sleep hygiene and habits.

4. The Mind in Sleep: Unlocking the Power of Dreams

Dream research is on the cusp of transformation. A deeper understanding of the purpose and significance of dreams may offer novel insights into mental health, emotional processing, and the mysteries of consciousness. The study of lucid dreaming, where individuals are aware they are dreaming, holds promise for exploring the boundaries of human consciousness.

5. Sleep as a Public Health Priority

As our understanding of the importance of sleep for overall well-being deepens, there is a growing recognition of the need to prioritize sleep as a public health imperative. Policies and interventions to improve sleep quality and address sleep disparities will likely gain momentum in the coming years.

The future of sleep science beckons with the promise of improving the lives of countless individuals grappling with sleep disturbances, whether they are plagued by insomnia, sleep apnea, or other sleep-related challenges. This evolving field is deepening our understanding of sleep and offering practical solutions that can enhance our sleep quality and overall well-being.

As we look ahead, the convergence of various disciplines—genetics, neuroscience, psychology, and technology—is poised to propel sleep research to new heights. Collaborative efforts among researchers and healthcare providers are accelerating the translation of scientific discoveries into tangible interventions for those in need.

6. Sleep as a Pillar of Public Health

The recognition of sleep as a fundamental pillar of public health is gaining momentum. Sleep disorders and chronic sleep deprivation are associated with a myriad of health issues, including cardiovascular disease, diabetes, obesity, and mental health disorders. This realization leads to increased advocacy for prioritizing sleep at societal and policy levels.

Public health campaigns and educational initiatives aim to raise awareness about sleep hygiene, consistent sleep schedules, and avoiding sleep-disrupting behaviours. The aim is to improve individual sleep and reduce the burden of sleep-related disorders on healthcare systems.

7. Holistic Approaches to Sleep

The future of sleep science embraces holistic approaches that recognize the interconnectedness of sleep with other aspects of our lives. Researchers are increasingly investigating the impact of lifestyle, diet, and physical activity on sleep quality. The promotion of comprehensive well-being is becoming integral to sleep interventions.

Yoga, mindfulness meditation, and relaxation techniques are integrated into sleep therapy programs, emphasizing the mind-body connection in sleep health. This holistic approach acknowledges that sleep cannot be isolated from our health and lifestyle choices.

8. Sleep and Aging

Understanding the relationship between sleep and ageing becomes paramount as our population ages. Older adults often face unique sleep challenges, including changes in sleep architecture, increased prevalence of sleep disorders, and age-related changes in circadian rhythms.

Research in this area explores strategies to improve sleep quality and promote healthy ageing. From tailored sleep interventions for older adults to the potential role of chronotherapy (adjusting the timing of interventions based on circadian rhythms), the future of sleep science is poised to enhance the sleep experiences of ageing populations.

9. Sleep and the Digital Age

The ubiquity of digital devices in our lives presents both opportunities and challenges for sleep. Ongoing research examines the impact of screen time, blue light exposure, and digital media consumption on sleep patterns. At the same time, innovative solutions are emerging to mitigate the adverse effects of technology on sleep.

Apps and wearable devices are designed to monitor sleep and promote healthy sleep habits. These digital tools offer customized recommendations for improving sleep hygiene and managing sleep disorders.

10. Interdisciplinary Collaboration

Perhaps one of the most promising aspects of the future of sleep science is the collaboration among diverse fields. The complexity of sleep necessitates interdisciplinary approaches that draw insights from biology, psychology, engineering, and social sciences.

Researchers are working together to unravel the intricate interactions between sleep and various domains of human life. This collaborative spirit fosters innovative solutions and a deeper understanding of sleep's role in our daily existence.

In Closing: A Bright Future for Sleep

As our journey through the intriguing landscape of the future of sleep science comes to a close, we stand at the precipice of a remarkable era—a time when the act of sleep transcends its conventional role as a nightly ritual and transforms into a boundless realm of discovery and enhanced well-being. The profound mysteries that have veiled the realm of sleep for so long are gradually giving way to the relentless pursuit of knowledge, igniting a beacon of hope for countless individuals who have yearned for the elusive embrace of restful slumber.

In this burgeoning epoch of sleep research, we find ourselves on the verge of a transformative renaissance—a renaissance that promises not only a deeper understanding of the multifaceted dimensions of sleep but also practical and personalized solutions that can revolutionize how we approach and experience the act of slumber.

The mysteries that once cloaked the enigma of sleep are gradually yielding to the collective efforts of researchers, scientists, and healthcare professionals who are driven by an insatiable curiosity to unearth the secrets hidden within the confines of our nighttime reverie. Our path is one of relentless inquiry and discovery, where each scientific breakthrough illuminates another facet of this intricate phenomenon.

As we gaze forward into this promising era, we are greeted by a tapestry of possibilities that can reshape our relationship with sleep. It is a time when sleep is not merely a passive state of rest but a dynamic arena where dreams are decoded, sleep disorders are deciphered, and the interplay between slumber and mental, emotional, and physical well-being is unravelled.

This impending age of sleep science invites us to explore the boundaries of what we thought we knew about rest and rejuvenation. It beckons us to embrace a holistic understanding of sleep, where every facet of our lives—our genetic makeup, daily routines, emotional landscapes, and technological interactions—interacts with and influences our nightly repose.

Sleep is no longer relegated to the sidelines in this epoch but emerges as a cornerstone of public health, a linchpin of cognitive function, and a conduit to emotional equilibrium. It stands as a sentinel guarding against the encroachment of chronic illness and an ally in the pursuit of longevity and vitality.

As we conclude this odyssey through the future of sleep science, we invite you to carry forth the torch of knowledge and curiosity. The journey continues, and with each passing day, we draw closer to a future where the embrace of restful slumber is not an elusive dream but a reality within our grasp. It is a future where sleep becomes a beacon of well-being, guiding us through the night and into the bright promise of each new day.

10

Embracing the Science of Sleep

Our journey through the pages of this book has been an exploration of the profound and intricate world of slumber. From the realms of dreams to the depths of the sleeping brain, we have delved into the science, the art, and the magic of sleep. As we conclude this enlightening voyage, we leave you with the major takeaway from our shared adventure—a newfound understanding of the significance of sleep and the compelling reasons to prioritize it for a healthier and more fulfilling life.

Throughout this book, we've embarked on a voyage of discovery, unravelling the enigma of sleep. We've uncovered the intricate workings of the sleep-wake cycle and the circadian rhythms that govern our lives. We've explored the stages of sleep and the architecture of our dreams. We've ventured into the realm of sleep disorders and their impact on well-being. We've examined the profound connections between sleep, mental health, and physical vitality. We've delved into the future of sleep science, where personalized interventions, technology, and holistic approaches promise to revolutionize how we understand and experience sleep.

At the heart of our journey lies a fundamental truth that cannot be overstated. Sleep is not a luxury; it is a necessity. It is the cornerstone of our physical, mental, and emotional well-being. Sleep is when our bodies heal, our minds rejuvenate, and our souls find solace. It is the canvas upon which our dreams are painted and the foundation of our waking lives.

The major takeaway from this exploration of sleep science is a simple yet profound realization: Sleep matters. It matters for your physical health, influencing everything from your immune system to your cardiovascular well-being. It matters for your mental health, as it plays a pivotal role in mood regulation and cognitive function. It matters for your emotional well-being, providing the respite and restoration needed to navigate life's challenges. It matters for your creativity, problem-solving abilities, and memory. It matters for your longevity and the quality of your life.

In the hurried pace of our modern lives, sleep often takes a backseat to the demands of work, family, and social commitments. We sacrifice sleep in pursuit of productivity and pay a steep price. Sleep deprivation exacts its toll on our bodies and minds, leaving us vulnerable to a host of health issues and impairing our ability to thrive.

Prioritizing Sleep: Your Path to a Healthier and More Fulfilling Life

As we conclude this journey, we urge you to take the wisdom of sleep science to heart. Prioritize sleep as an essential pillar of your well-being. Create a sleep-friendly environment in your bedroom, embrace good sleep hygiene practices, and nurture a consistent sleep routine. Seek help if you struggle with sleep disorders, for there are effective interventions that can make a profound difference in your life.

But beyond the practical strategies, we encourage you to cultivate a mindset that values sleep as a precious gift that restores, replenishes, and renews you each night. Sleeping is not a luxury but an investment in your health and vitality. Sleep is not a passive state but a vibrant, dynamic part of your life.

As we leave you with these parting words, remember that you hold the key to unlocking the secrets of restful nights and energized days. You can prioritize sleep as a foundation for better health, greater resilience, and a more fulfilling life. The science of sleep has illuminated the path; it is now up to you to walk it.

In the chapters of your life that follow, may you embrace the wisdom of slumber and awaken each day with renewed vigour, clarity, and purpose. May you savour the richness of your dreams and the refreshing embrace of restful nights. May you prioritize sleep not as an afterthought but as a profound act of self-care—a testament to your commitment to a life well-lived, one night at a time.

About the Author

Grace Fields, the author of this book, is a passionate advocate for happiness and well-being. Her journey is rooted in a profound appreciation for the transformative power of joy, and she is dedicated to sharing her insights with others. With a solid background in psychology and a deep love for personal growth, Grace effortlessly marries her knowledge with a compassionate writing style, offering readers valuable and practical guidance.

Having authored her first book, "The Science and Secrets of Lasting Happiness," Grace Fields brings a wealth of experience and wisdom to her latest work. Her writing is not just a profession but a heartfelt mission to help individuals discover the beauty of the present moment, forge meaningful connections, and nurture their overall well-being. Drawing from her own life experiences and a deep reservoir of research in positive psychology, mindfulness, and self-care, Grace's work is a beacon of inspiration.

Grace underscores the significance of gratitude, resilience, and self-compassion in her writing as transformative forces in our lives. Through her books and writings, she equips readers with the tools they need to navigate life's challenges, encouraging them to chart their path to happiness. Grace Fields is not just an author but a guiding light for those seeking a more joyful and fulfilling existence.